SLEEP W]

LIVE BETTER

How to Eliminate Stress and Stop Overthinking at Night. Change Your Sleeping Habits, Increase Your Productivity w/ Positive Energy During the Day and Declutter Your Mind

By

Gary Foster

The information in the following pages is broadly considered a truthful and accurate account of facts and as such, any inattention, use, or misuse of the information in question by the reader will render any resulting actions solely under their purview. There are no scenarios in which the publisher or the original author of this work can be in any fashion deemed liable for any hardship or damages that may befall them after undertaking information described herein.

Additionally, the information in the following pages is intended only for informational purposes and should thus be thought of as universal. As befitting its nature, it is presented without assurance regarding its prolonged validity or interim quality. Trademarks that are mentioned are done without written consent and can in no way be considered an endorsement from the trademark holder.

Table of Content

Introduction

Sleep is a complex and active process of physiological restoration. It is the condition of the body and mind in which the nervous system is in a restorative mode; the eyes are closed, and consciousness is temporarily suspended. It naturally occurs as a state of altered consciousness, in which there is a decreased ability to react to external stimuli. In this condition, activities of the senses are inhibited, and almost all of the voluntary muscles are inactive.

Sleep is a biological state of rest. During sleep, the brain stays active while most of the body's organ systems are in a state of increased repair and maintenance at the cellular level. It is an established biological need. About one-third of our existence consists of sleep. It is essential for maintaining productivity throughout the day. Without restorative sleep, a person cannot learn, create, and communicate at the optimal level. A few skips of a good night's rest can cause substantial stress for the body, which can potentially lead to a major mental and physical breakdown.

History And Background Of Sleep

Long before research established scientific facts about it, sleep was considered to be a passive state in which the brain becomes "inactive" or "switched off". Throughout history, sleep patterns and ideas pertaining to it have evolved, but the need for this "sweet balm" that soothes and restores our body after a long day of work and play has not changed. To this day, many sleep scientists are still studying and making sense of the mystery of this process. There are still a lot of gray areas in the field of sleep, but observations and studies made throughout history have nevertheless contributed to further understanding the inner workings of the body during this significant biological process.

In 600-800 B.C., segmented sleep was largely the norm for centuries. This means that two sleep periods in a day was common, and it was a period of prayer, thinking, reflecting on dreams, drinking ale, and visiting neighbors at night.

In 450-500 B.C., the earliest documented sleep theory was written by Alcmaeon. He stated that sleep was a loss of consciousness that occurred when blood drained from the vessels on the body surface. His study resulted in further observation and experimentation about sleep.

Around 400 B.C., a new theory was suggested that bodies tend to feel cool to the touch when people sleep as blood goes to the inner regions of the body. This was recorded in Corpus Hippocraticum, a collection of medical writings largely attributed to Hippocrates. Also, the concept of circadian rhythm, and internally controlled body process that repeats itself every 24 hours, was first recorded by Androsthenes, the scribe of Alexander the Great.

In 350 B.C., sleep was viewed as a necessary time of physical recovery. Aristotle theorized that sleep was caused directly by warm vapors rising from the stomach to the heart, which was believed at that time to be the organ that controls consciousness. This was also the reason used to explain why people feel sleepy after having a meal.

Around 162 A.D., it was discovered that the brain controlled consciousness. Galen experimented on the brain and refuted Aristotle's claim.

In 1584, Aristotle's theory that warm vapors from the stomach were rising to the heart during digestion that caused sleep, was promoted by Thomas Cogan. He suggested that meat, milk, and wine produced a lot of these "warm vapors" more readily than any other food item.

In the Renaissance era, theories related to sleep and wakefulness began to emerge. Some scientists and philosophers believed that sleep was caused by oxygen or blood deprivation in the brain. Others believed that toxins build up in the body during the state of wakefulness, and then get flushed out during sleep. Still, others thought it was an inhibitory reflex that shut off the body and caused sleep.

During the Age of Enlightenment, dreams were viewed as significant and sacred. Interpretation and recording of dreams became a trend, especially among the intellectual class. Alfred Maury and Marquis d'Hervey de Saint-Denis were prominent among those who recorded their dreams daily, studied them, and interpreted them.

In the Industrial Age, the bedroom was regarded as a strictly personal area. Also, sleeping beyond seven to eight hours a day was viewed negatively as lazy.

In the 1900s, scientists began to discover that the brain, not the sun or stomach gases, controlled sleep and wakefulness. The science of sleep medicine was also born. In 1939, Nathaniel Kleitman published recordings of his years of investigative and experimental research in Sleep and Wakefulness, which is regarded as a milestone in the study of sleep.

In 1970, the first sleep center (the laboratory where studies of sleep and diagnoses of sleep disorders can be properly conducted) was established at Stanford University. The Association of Sleep Disorders was also founded. In 1983, studies made by Allan Rechtschaffen and his colleagues revealed that sleep deprivation results in serious health problems and even death. Many studies are highlighting the importance of sleep. Even so, many people in this decade find it difficult to manage their hectic schedules to accommodate enough sleep time to recover properly from their daily lives.

Chapter 1: Know Sleep

What Is Sleep?

Despite all the studies that have taken place, the subject of sleep still remains quite a mystery to us. When we imagine someone sleeping, we imagine this person being still, all their muscles relaxed, and breathing deeply. We tend not to think of this as being a very active phase of our day. However, as we learn more about sleep, we will see that those who are asleep can be very active, both physically and mentally. Their brain waves are active, and their body is performing thousands of micro-tasks.

How Does Our Body Know When To Go To Sleep?

Our body has its own internal clock. This clock can be influenced by several factors, such as natural daylight and our own man-made routines. This internal clock is referred to as our circadian clock, and just like our day on Earth, it has roughly a 24-hour cycle. This 'clock' is actually a bundle of brain cells, called neurons, which are located in a specific region within the hypothalamus of the brain. This area of our brain is responsible for regulating essential body functions such as body temperature, blood pressure, heart rate, hormone production, and telling us when we need to eat. The circadian clock also lets us know when we need to go to sleep.

Your circadian clock is mainly influenced by the light and darkness of the day. When light stimulates the receptors at the back of the eye, a message is sent to the brain, which then recognizes that it is daytime and that the body should be in a state of awareness.

During our waking hours, our body creates a neurotransmitter called adenosine. Adenosine has a depressant effect on the central nervous system, helping to quieten and suppress it, preparing the body for sleep. The amount of adenosine in your body increases each hour that you are awake.

When the light begins to fade, the brain then releases a hormone called melatonin. The body responds to the presence of melatonin by reducing body temperature and causing us to feel tired and drowsy, indicating to us that it is time to sleep.

Therefore, a combination of increased adenosine and melatonin will trigger the feeling of tiredness, making us want to go to sleep. During the night, the levels of these chemicals will decrease, so that we will awaken and feel active with the increase of daylight that surrounds us.

Stages Of Sleep

For the purpose of simplicity, we can break the stages of sleep down into four. The first three are termed as non-REM (non-Rapid Eye Movement), and the fourth is the REM stage.

Stage 1 is the initial sleep stage when your muscles start to relax, your eye movements begin to slow, heart rate becomes regular, blood pressure begins to drop, and your breathing slows down. You find yourself drifting in and out of sleep. It is very easy to waken from this stage of sleep.

As you progress through to Stage 2, you enter the light sleep stage. Your brain waves gradually become slower, eye movements stop, heart rate becomes slower, and your metabolism begins to slow, your body temperature decreases. Your body is preparing itself for a deeper sleep.

In Stage 3, your eyes stop moving, and your brain waves have slowed down and entered the delta wave frequency. Waking from this stage of sleep is quite hard, and if disturbed, you could feel disorientated for a short while afterward. Stage 3 is a very important stage of sleep for the body physically. During this phase of a deep sleep, the body repairs and renews itself. This includes repairing and replacing tissue and bone, synthesizing essential hormones, and strengthening the immune system.

REM (Rapid Eye Movement) sleep is probably the best-known stage of sleep. This is the stage in which we dream. Our brain waves become active again as if we are awake. However, our muscles remain completely still, almost as if we are paralyzed. Not only do our brain waves stir, and eyes begin to move once again, our heart rate and blood pressure also begin to increase, so does our temperature. Our breathing is less shallow and becomes more rapid. We tend to enter this phase of sleep after we have been sleeping for around 90 minutes.

These stages of sleep are then repeated. We can enter the REM stage between 3 to 5 times each night, and each time, the REM stage increases in length. The first REM stage may only last 5 to 10 minutes while the last may continue for up to an hour.

There is a natural pattern to sleep, and should it be broken, we feel disorientated, find it hard to fall back to sleep, and subsequent essential processes that should take place don't get the chance to be carried out.

From this basic overview, we can see how important sleep is for the body to rest, repair, and renew. Therefore, disturbed or reduced sleep can have a huge negative impact on, not only our positive outlook but our health and wellbeing also.

How Much Sleep Do You Need?

For adults over the age of 18 years, a full night of sleep should last between 7 to 9 hours.

This means that we need to allow up to 9 hours in our day for this resting time.

If we do not pay attention to the hours of sleep that we get, the sleep debt soon mounts up, and it's not something you can 'payback'.

For those who sleep less during the week and sleep more at weekends to make up the lost hours, unfortunately, when it comes to sleep loss, it's not that simple. Each time you lose sleep, your body reacts automatically, going into a stress response. We're not talking about complete sleep deprivation here, or even a few months of little sleep before our body triggers the stress response. Problems can start with just missing a full night's sleep now and again. It all adds up, and all add stress to the body.

Taking more hours to sleep during the weekend's messes with your circadian rhythm and makes it harder to get back into a sleep routine in time for the working week once more. Having regular sleep and wake times is the best way to make sure that you keep your sleep pattern healthy.

We have only looked briefly at just a few physical side effects of sleep deprivation, and perhaps, as one who suffers from insomnia, you may have identified with some of them already.

Personally, I can relate to the subject of weight gain, and I discovered, after years of my weight fluctuating, that having a regular sleeping pattern helps restore my weight to where it should be.

The list of side effects written here is not a scaremongering tactic to make sure you sleep early every night – they are true researched facts, and I have included them in order to broaden the concept that sleep is not merely time to be lazy and chill out, but it has a proper physiological function within our body, and we cannot function healthily without it.

Sleep is an essential component for gaining positivity in life – whether it be physical or mental wellbeing that contributes to generating this positivity, and as mentioned before, it tends to be a part of our lifestyle that we overlook.

When we are ill, on whatever level, we look for a cause. We look at the whys and the remedies. We look towards our lifestyle, our exercise, our diet, or daytime stress levels. We seldom relate our ill-health to the lack of or poor quality of sleep.

The National Sleep Foundation, based in America, regularly conduct several polls and have found that even though adults need between 7 and 9 hours of sleep a night to maintain their health, 40% of adults were found to be having less than 7 hours of sleep during the week, and more alarmingly, it isn't just adults that are not getting the correct amount of sleep.

As many as 29% of 12 to 14-year old was getting less than 7 hours of sleep, and even more worryingly, 56% of 15 to 17-year old was also sleeping less than 7 hours a night. Considering children of these ages should still be having at least 9 hours of sleep a night, this is worrying information, and is no doubt having a negative impact on their physical and mental health. There have been several studies carried out showing that, not surprisingly, a lack of sleep has a detrimental effect on the academic performance, behavior, and weight of children.

Below is a table showing the hours of sleep for each age category, as recommended by the National Sleep Foundation.

Age	Recommended Hours of Sleep
0 – 3 months	14 – 17 hours
4 – 11 months	12 – 15 hours
1 – 2 years	11 – 14 hours
3 – 5 years	10 – 13 hours
6 – 13 years	9 – 11 hours
14 – 17 years	8 – 10 hours
18 – 25 years	7 – 9 hours
26 – 64 years	7 – 9 hours
65 years plus	7 – 8 hours

Chapter 2: Benefits of sleep

There are certain people who tend to ignore the benefits of having an adequate sleep. For them, it is only part of the usual routine. If you look into the matter deeply, you are lucky if you don't have any trouble sleeping.

Following a healthy sleeping habit affects your body in a variety of ways and causes the following health benefits:

1. Longer lifespan. Aside from making you healthier, having a sufficient sleep affects the quality of your life. It makes you feel better and gives you a lighter aura on how you will go about your daily routine. Upon waking up, you will feel refreshed and energized, which is the opposite when you lack sleep, or you overslept.

2. Better memory. Your mind works as you sleep. It consolidates the skills that you have learned during your waking hours.

For example, you are trying to learn a new language. Your mind will help you retain the information as you sleep. Upon waking up, it is easier to remember the words that you have already encountered, continue the learning process, and memorize more unfamiliar words and phrases faster.

Aside from consolidating memories, your brain also restructures or reorganizes as you sleep. This will help in spurring your creativity or form ideas, especially if you are in the middle of thinking about what to paint, draw, or write. There are studies, which found out that the emotional factors of a person's memory, are strengthened by having a sufficient amount of sleep. This is what ignites your creative blood and ideas upon waking up.

3. Perform better at school. In 2010, the Journal Sleep found out that children aged 10-16, who suffer from interrupted breathing while sleeping, such as sleep apnea and snoring, are more prone to having difficulties in learning and focusing. This had a great effect on how they performed in school. It is okay to sacrifice sleep once in a while when you are trying to meet a deadline or review for an exam, but make sure that you don't do this all the time.

Lack of sleep has opposite effects on adults and kids. Adults tend to lose energy and feel sleepy. Kids show symptoms that are similar to those who are suffering from ADHD. Kids who lack sleep are more likely to get hyperactive, impulsive, and inattentive.

4. Reduce the risk of having inflammation. People who get less than six hours of sleep at night tend to have higher blood levels of proteins that cause inflammation as compared to those who get sufficient rest. When this

happens, you are placing yourself at a high risk of developing diseases, such as diabetes, stroke, heart problems, and arthritis. This will also affect your appearance and will make you look older at a faster rate.

5. Decrease your stress levels. It is only natural to face various stressful factors in your everyday life. Higher stress level makes you susceptible to cardiovascular diseases. There are many ways to battle out stress, and one of the most effective techniques is to sleep and get sufficient rest. This will clear your mind and give you a refreshed outlook. This way, you will have an easier time facing your troubles and think of ways about how to counter these.

6. Improved performance for athletes. Having a sufficient amount of rest will boost your stamina, which is important when you are involved in physically draining activities. This will make you a better athlete because you can move with more confidence and will not easily get fatigued. This is actually a requirement for those who are involved in sports, such as football, tennis, and swimming.

7. Healthy weight. If you are planning to lose weight, make sure that you get sufficient sleep. Many dieters feel hungrier when they lose sleep. This is due to the fact that the same sectors of the brain control sleep and metabolism. When a person is sleepy, the hormones that

cause the hunger sensation go up in the blood. As a result, it boosts the person's appetite, and he/she craves for food.

8. Happier mood. Lack of sleep can make you feel moody. Enough rest makes your emotions more stable, decreases your anxiety, and makes you feel happier. It helps improve your mood so that you don't get irritated and angry easily. No matter how busy you are, you need to find a balance and get enough rest every day. If you are sleeping too much during the weekends, this means that you aren't getting sufficient rest for the rest of the week. This is not healthy. You cannot make up for lost sleep by sleeping too much for a day or two.

9. Healthy skin. During the first three hours of your deep slumber, the body is at its most active in producing growth hormone that is important in the skin repair process. The following two hours is the phase when rapid eye movement (REM) begins. This is when the body produces melatonin, a kind of hormone that acts as an antioxidant. Most REM sleep happens during the last three hours. This is when the skin's temperature reaches its lowest, causing the muscles to relax and allowing the skin to recover. You need to experience each phase every night as you sleep, so your skin needs at least nine hours of sleep in order to become healthier.

10. Stronger immune system. There are studies, which proved that people who slept adequately are less likely to get sick as compared to those who frequently lose sleep.

11. Lower risk of injury. There are a lot of reported accidents that happened due to drivers who fell asleep or were sleepy while on the road. In the US alone, it is estimated that one out of five car accidents that happen in a day is caused by drowsy driving. There are many other kinds of accidents that you can avoid if you are alert because you've got enough rest. These mishaps include falling, slipping, accidentally cutting yourself, and many more.

12. Better sex life. Men who often get insufficient sleep have lower testosterone levels than those who follow a healthy sleeping routine. Your sex life will also likely suffer for the mere reason that you are quite tired due to lack of sleep. It is worse when you are only on the dating level, and you often fall asleep in the midst of a movie, or you look uninterested while having a dinner date.

It all boils down to balance. No matter how busy you are, you must always remind yourself that sleep is essential.

Chapter 3: The Importance of Having Adequate Sleep

Science has proven that those who sleep and rise early and get a good night's rest tend to be happier and more successful in life as compared to those who miss out on a good night's sleep on a regular basis. Let us dig deeper into the importance of sleeping well by listing out the many reasons why you must build a healthy sleep routine:

Provides Your Body With Enough Rest And Improves Your Energy Levels

Sleep is the time when your body relaxes after a full day of toil, and you worked out, and torn muscles get to rejuvenate during that time. This is the time when different growth hormones are also released in your body to repair the worn-out muscles and rehabilitate them. If you keep pushing your body to work throughout the night as well and that too on a regular basis, it explains why you feel so exhausted always.

Not only your body, but your mind also needs to rest after an entire day of thinking actively. The truth is, your mind is still working when you rest and sleep, but the activity does slow down. It works on areas other than analytical thinking, planning, brainstorming, and active decision-making, which gives it a chance to unwind and relax.

This explains why you find it easier to comfortably leave your bed and feel fresh after a good night's rest. According to a survey by the 'Better Sleep Council', 32% Americans believe that one of the best benefits of getting a solid's night rest is their increased physical and mental energy. Sufficient sleep helps stabilize the hormones in your body, which also helps you make healthier eating choices. This consequently steadies the sugar levels in your body, which provides you with sustained energy throughout the day.

Improves Your Heart Health And Blood Pressure

If you are worried about having poor heart health since it runs in your family, start improving your sleep routine. A study shows that a solid night's sleep is a great way to safeguard your heart against cardiac arrest. The study examined the sleep habits of over 52,000 Norwegian people and observed that those who sleep less, and experience insomnia have a 30 to 45% greater risk of experiencing a heart attack as compared to those who sleep well throughout the night. A lack of sleep often leads to high blood pressure as well as hormonal changes in your body, both of which pave the way for a cardiac arrest.

When you sleep well, these issues resolve, and your heart health improves, which then reduces your likelihood of experiencing heart-related problems.

Also, studies show people who get less sleep have 80% more chances of experiencing hypertension (high blood pressure) than those who sleep properly through the night. Deep sleep helps stabilize your blood pressure as it lowers down during that time. This regulates your heartbeat and blood pressure, which helps you overcome hypertension.

Improved Emotional Wellbeing

It should not come as a surprise to you that sleeping well does cheer you up. Compare your mood and emotional wellbeing when you sleep well through the night to a time when you keep tossing and turning on your bed the entire night. The answer shows a marked improvement in your cheerfulness and your ability to think clearly.

Ample sleep improves the production of mood, improving hormones such as serotonin and dopamine, which boost your confidence, energy, and happiness, helping you stay energetic, happy, calm, and enthusiastic throughout the day.

Also, when you feel happy, you stay positive, which improves your ability to think clearly and make rational decisions. A study by the National Sleep Foundation also shows that there exists a complicated and robust association between depression and insomnia. People who have insomnia have 10 times more likelihood of suffering from depression as compared to healthy sleepers. One reason behind this is that often when you don't sleep, you rehash the past memories or think about future concerns, which can often open old wounds or make you too concerned about the future, respectively. This increases your tensions and paves the way for depression.

Fortunately, these issues can be combatted successfully, especially by improving your sleep routine. When you rest properly through the night, you allow your body to stabilize the hormonal issues, which improves your mood and consequently the quality of your life.

Moreover, a survey by the National Sleep Foundation found out that over 85% participants of the study who received insufficient sleep throughout the night complained that this adversely affected their temper and mood; 72% reported that a lack of sleep impacts their household responsibilities and family life, and 68% stated that it negatively influenced their social lives. This happens because a lack of sleep also increases the levels of cortisol in your body, which is the notorious stress hormone. The more the cortisol in your body, the more you feel stressed out. That said, getting a good night's rest daily helps lower the cortisol levels and improves your mood.

Helps You Eat Healthy And Manage Your Weight

If you are having a hard time managing your weight, pay attention to your sleep routine. It is likely you stay awake for the major part of the night, and this is a major reason why you do not have healthy eating habits and cannot lose weight successfully.

Experts suggest that skipping sleep is often the culprit that keeps you from losing weight easily because it messes with your metabolism. People who do not sleep well mostly have low levels of 'leptin', which is the satiety hormone. Low levels of leptin mean you feel satiated slowly and eat more to feel satisfied.

Also, a lack of sleep promotes the production of 'ghrelin', which is the hunger hormone, so not sleeping enough means you feel hungrier throughout the day and eat more. This is why you are always feeling ravenous, particularly for sugar-laden foods.

Studies show that healthy sleepers who get at least 6 to 8 hours of sleep on average are better able to follow their weight loss regimen primarily because their ghrelin and leptin levels are stabilized.

Also, since sleeping well increases your energy levels and ability to think rationally, you are able to feel fresher and make healthier food choices during the day and stay on the right track when it comes to losing weight.

Reduces Risk Of Suffering From Diabetes

Inadequate sleep over a long period can make you develop high insulin resistance, which is a precursor to suffering from diabetes. Research has also discovered that the quality and duration of your sleep affect the levels of hormones involved in triggering diabetes; therefore, if you sleep less, you are likely to become more prone to acquiring diabetes or pre-diabetes. Improving your sleep routine is definitely a way to overcome these problems and stay fitter.

Reinforces Your Immune System

Research shows that healthy sleepers have a better immune system than the ones who complain of never sleeping enough. A study in Archives of Internal Medicine from 2009 shows that those who sleep fewer than 7 hours at night have 3 times more chances of suffering from common cold as compared to those who sleep longer than that. If you want a strong, healthy immune system that kicks off diseases efficiently from your system, have an adequate sleep.

Improves Your Skin

Yes, 'beauty sleep' does exist, and it is exactly what you need to have a healthy, supple, and glowing skin. Restorative, deep sleep improves the production of your body cells, which reduces the breakdown of skin proteins and helps your skin repair the damage it goes through, which improves its health and condition.

Improves Your Love Life And Relationships

Studies show that when you sleep less, you become more irritable towards your partner and even everyone else during the day, which only negatively affects your relationships.

In addition, a lack of sleep makes you grumpy, stressed out, and annoyed, which decreases your ability to stay calm with people and make better decisions. This does take a toll on your love life and other important relationships.

Fortunately, this can be reversed by improving your sleep routine. Healthy sleepers tend to have a better marriage and build healthy relationships in life as compared to insomniacs as the former is more composed, calmer, energetic, and happier in life.

A study in 2011 shows that improved sleep also improves your sex drive and consequently your sex life. This can be because a good night's rest improves your energy levels and enthusiasm. Also, it boosts testosterone levels in men, which improves their libido. Therefore, when you sleep well daily, you are likely to enjoy a better sex life with your partner, which also improves your love/ marital life.

Improved Brainpower

A healthy sleep routine does wonder to your brainpower. A night of deep REM sleep helps reinforce the important pieces of information you noticed during the day and creates long-term memories.

Further, during your sleep, your brain discards meaningless information from your mind to prevent information overload. Your brain also clears toxins out of your system when you are asleep, which improves your brain health and overall cognition.

Additionally, a good night's rest improves your brain's plasticity and connectivity. Plasticity is required for improved learning and reinforcing your memory. There is plenty of evidence, which suggests how a lack of sleep can cause problems with your working memory and hampers your ability to process information. If you wish to have a sharper memory and improved cognition, just focus on getting enough sleep.

Reduces Likelihood Of Acquiring Cancer

A study in the journal titled 'Cancer' discovered that those who sleep 6 or fewer hours at night have a staggering 50% risk of acquiring colorectal adenomas, which is a precursor to having cancerous tumors as compared to all those who clock in at a minimum of 7 hours every night. Another study shows that a lack of sleep increases your chances of suffering from colon cancer.

Improves Your Focus And Productivity

Naturally, when you rest well, you focus better on your work, which improves your work performance and reduces slip-ups. This increases your productivity and opens up more opportunities for growth and advancement in your career so you can easily accomplish your professional goals.

All these positive changes in your life help you live better and feel good about yourself. Also, a study published in 2007 shows that adequate sleep helps you cope successfully with chronic pain as it relaxes your joints and muscles and improves your ability to manage pain.

Now that you are aware of all the reasons why you must sleep well, let us share with you the ways you can implement to improve your sleep routine.

Chapter 4: How Lack of Sleep Affects Your Emotional Health

We all know that lack of sleep might be the reason behind our snapping at someone, but most of us are not fully aware of how strongly sleep deprivation hurts our emotional wellbeing. Lack of sleep affects our mental health, sense of wellbeing, performance, mindset, and outlook, as well as our relationships.

Sleep Deprivation Makes You More Impulsive And Reactive

When you don't get enough sleep, you're likely to be more emotionally reactive. Your actions will be more intense and impulsive. You might find yourself losing your temper with your kids, fighting with your partner, or lashing out at coworkers. These situations are not fun, and they don't contribute to the quality of our relationships.

It's not just about being grumpy. We go further by beating ourselves up for not being in control of our emotions, which leaves us exhausted, drained, and critical of ourselves.

If you don't sleep well just for one night, you end up being testier and less in control of your reactions. And when it comes to chronic sleep deprivation, these kinds of negative outbursts can become an everyday occurrence.

Science still doesn't know all about the connection between our emotions and sleep, but there are interesting discoveries about how lack of sleep affects the emotional centers of the brain, making us impulsive, irritable, frustrated, and angry.

Many types of diagnostics, including EEG, brain scanning, and magnet resonance, show the same thing: sleep deprivation increases activity in the amygdala, the center of the brain responsible for rapid emotional response. This part is responsible for controlling our immediate emotional reactions. When you lack sleep, the amygdala goes into overdrive. It's the same as if you were driving with broken brakes. That's why you become highly reactive to situations.

However, it's not only our negative emotions that are increased when we lack sleep. Sleep deprivation makes us more reactive to all emotions, positive ones too.

Not only is the amygdala in overdrive mode, but a lack of sleep hinders communication between the amygdala and the prefrontal cortex, another part of the brain responsible for the regulation of our emotions.

The prefrontal cortex is responsible for many complex tasks, among them being regulation of our impulsiveness. It controls and calms our impulsive reactions.

When you don't get enough sleep, the prefrontal cortex can't function as well, and you become less thoughtful and react more impulsively.

Life is full of emotionally charged experiences. They are stored in our memories, and sleep plays a significant role in processing them. REM sleep is crucial for processing unpleasant and painful memories and helps us to ease the pain this kind of memories can cause. Besides that, sleep helps your brain to bounce back to emotional balance, so this rest is crucial for your emotional and mental health. When you don't get enough REM sleep, your mind doesn't experience these therapeutic benefits.

You Start To Have A Negative Outlook

It's not surprising that lack of sleep contributes to a negative mindset. Sleep deprivation makes us focus on the negative, and keeps our mind stuck, going over negative thoughts again and again. It's called repetitive negative thinking. Repetitive negative thoughts make you feel bad and prevent you from performing well. They are hard to control when you are tired, and they can contribute to the development of depression and anxiety.

We may all know this from experience, but there are also scientific studies that have proven that sleep-deprived people are more focused on the negative, have more repetitive negative thoughts, and have difficulty in controlling them than their rested counterparts. The more tired you are, the harder it is to control negative thoughts and shift your mind away from them. Being stuck in the cycle of negative thinking is a truly bad experience, but it's exactly what happens when you chronically lack sleep.

You Become Anxious And Concerned About The Future

Sleep deprivation also makes us worry more. If you are prone to worry in general, it becomes much worse when you're sleep-deprived, recent studies show. When you are trapped in this negative cycle, the future doesn't seem safe or bright.

Interesting research conducted by scientists at the University of California Berkeley shows that sleep deprivation increases anticipatory anxiety, the kind that has you worrying about the future. It also worsens symptoms of regular anxiety and can contribute to developing an anxiety disorder. So, if you, in general, tend to worry, make sure you get plenty of rest to maintain a healthy emotional balance and avoid developing mental health issues connected to anxiety.

You Are Less Grateful And Lack of Empathy

Sleep deprivation directly affects our sense of appreciation. Since gratefulness is a boost for positive emotions and nurtures our relationships, it's not surprising that we are less connected to our partners when we lack sleep. A study was conducted to examine the connection between the amount and quality of sleep and a sense of gratefulness. Unsurprisingly, people in the sleep-deprived group could remember fewer things they are thankful for than those who slept through the night.

Interestingly, the study found that it's enough for one of the partners to be short of sleep for both to have a diminished sense of gratefulness. So, if you don't sleep well, not only do you feel less grateful for your partner, but he also has less appreciation for you.

When sleep-deprived, we are less able to show empathy (recognizing and understanding others' emotions). We can't accurately recognize emotions in others. Of course, it affects our relationships, too. We are less able to walk in another's shoes, to see things from a different perspective, and to connect.

Gratefulness, appreciation for other people, empathy, and self-awareness are all vital parts of one's emotional intelligence. Sleep deprivation diminishes them, often weakening our most important relationships—couples who lack sleep fight more and solve problems less successfully than rested people. According to research, if just one of the partners lacks sleep, it's enough for conflicts to increase.

It's Not The Same For Men And Women

Like many other things in life, men and women experience sleep deprivation differently. It refers to emotional impact, too. When they don't get enough quality rest, women experience more anger, resentment, and depression in the morning than men. Women's brains, in general, spend more energy than men. That's perhaps due to women's ability to multitask. This expanded spending means that women need more restorative sleep for healthy brain functioning. When they don't get it, emotional issues can arise more often and sooner than in men.

Obviously, sleeping well and enough is crucial for your mental health, your inner balance, relationships, and emotional well-being.

Chapter 5: Problems of not Getting Enough Sleep and Correctly

Insomnia

At the core, insomnia is a condition wherein someone has difficulty falling asleep and maintaining sleep.

You, as an adult, might have experienced this a few times in the past, especially during stressful times or before a big planned event in your life. These short phased and finite periods of sleeplessness characterize acute insomnia.

On the other hand, there are those who have been suffering from this condition over extended periods of time. This could be because of traumatic events or biological reasons. This is known as chronic insomnia.

Whether it's acute or chronic, one thing is always constant: your body doesn't get enough rest when you suffer from insomnia. It affects your day, mood, and performance.

In today's hectic lifestyle, Insomnia has been considered as the most common sleeping disorder in the United States. More than 25 million people suffer from either acute or chronic insomnia.

Symptoms

It's difficult to tell if you have insomnia because the symptoms could easily be passed off as being tired or stressed or just the simple cause of the daily grind. With that being said, it's important to notice a pattern in these signs.

- Inability to fall asleep. Despite having the chance to lie down to get some rest, you can't seem to coerce your body into thinking that it is time to recuperate. You could either be worried about something or you feel that you still have something to do.

- Interrupted sleep. After successfully entering your first few non-REM cycles of sleep, you tend to wake up, feeling tired and irritated at the lack of rest. Even without external stimuli or disturbances, you manage to wake yourself before you arrive at your REM cycles.

- Waking up unnecessarily early. This is when you can no longer go back to sleep once you end your current cycle. You feel that you have to get started with the day despite not having enough rest.

- Errors in memorization and focus. Because of the lack of rest, you find it hard to place your mind at the right frequency needed for the work ahead of you. You also have problems remembering tasks, things, and even people.

Besides these, there could be other symptoms connected to insomnia. You could be making a lot of mistakes at work or even worse, committing accidents while you're out and about.

The problem with undiagnosed cases of insomnia is that people tend to disregard these symptoms and just assume that they will disappear the moment that they're able to go home and get some more sleep.

This is how acute insomnia becomes chronic. Without any medical or therapeutic intervention, these symptoms just end up prolonging your suffering.

Treatment

The first step to treating insomnia is to accept that there is a pattern of sleeplessness in your daily routine. You have to stop assuming that it will all go away if you had a whole night to yourself or when the weekend sets in.

When you've recognized this pattern, don't try to solve the problem on your own. Mention it to your physician and ask for advice. Should they be knowledgeable about sleeping disorders, they may be able to make some recommendations.

This is important because you're only halfway there. Now that you know there is a problem, the following step is to find the cause of the problem. It could be simple anxiety or something much worse. Knowing what causes insomnia allows doctors to make the right recommendations.

- Medical Problems. You might already be suffering from something else, which makes you unable to sleep. Interestingly, several other sicknesses entail insomnia as one of their symptoms. Examples of these are kidney disorders, Parkinson's disease, asthma, and even cancer. You may need to go through medical examinations to find what's ailing your sleep patterns.

- Depression, anxiety and stress. These are the most common causes of insomnia, especially in chronic cases. Most people are worried about a number of things, or they could be emotionally scarred from a traumatic event for a long time. They could also be suffering from chronic stress, which causes your body to feel like it is under threat despite already lying down on your bed.

- Medication. You could already be trying to solve another problem with your body by taking medicine. Your doctor will almost always ask and check your records if they've prescribed you anything that will cause you to lose sleep. It's also a good idea to take a look at your vitamins and supplements and ask about them. In other rare cases, even birth control pills have been found to cause insomnia in some women.

- Other sleep problems. At the core, insomnia could be a symptom or a disorder in itself. Sometimes, it also means you have other sleeping problems that require additional attention. You could be suffering from sleep apnea or jetlag or even a deviation from your circadian rhythm.

Jet Lag

What is just considered as a side-effect of flying through different time zones could be something that drastically affects the quality of your sleep.

Jet lag is a condition wherein you cannot sleep well and experience other discomforts when you pass through several time zones. Frequent flyers talk about this condition when they make several breaks through different continents, each with their own time zones.

People who suffer from jet lag usually find it hard to sleep or become really sleepy at inappropriate times of the country in which they've arrived. Because of the different time zones, you could still be greeted by the morning sun after a twelve-hour flight that took off in the early morning.

When your body expects it to be nighttime with the absence of sunlight but is greeted hours later by the same sunlight despite a long amount of time passing, then it's bound to cause an imbalance within your natural rhythm. This could lead to the following things:

- Irritability

- Fatigue

- Loss of Focus

- Lethargy

- Headaches

- Digestive problems

- Insomnia

Should you experience these symptoms after a long flight, that means your body is reeling from the effects of the changing zones. This means you need to get quality sleep in order to reset your functions.

Treatment

In most cases, jet lag serves as a temporary drawback to the wonders of travel. Give yourself a day of rest, and your body will have completely adjusted to the new time zone.

With that being said, there are a few more remedies available to help you better adapt to this phenomenon:

- If you're staying in a new country for several days, give yourself a few days of rest, equal to the number of time zones you'll be crossing. If you're only staying abroad for a short while, try to maintain your original sleep schedule and put up with the initial discomforts of your destination. It's better than adjusting once more when you come back home.

- Adapt to your Destination. If your destination is several hours ahead, train yourself to sleep the same time the people their sleep, even if you're not yet there. Use an international clock to keep track of the time differences as you adjust your sleeping patterns. You won't be shocked by jet lag as much if you've been changing your sleep schedule before your plan leaves.

- Avoid in-flight alcohol and caffeine. These substances will only either give you a rush or a down, which are both unnecessary as you pass through different time zones. These will only tarnish the quality of sleep you get while you're in-flight.

- Use Melatonin. Think of this as one of the few cases where a sleeping aid is necessary. As you approach the time zone of your destination, you need to coincide with your sleep pattern with theirs. This may be difficult, especially when you're going through a large time difference. Melatonin will help ease your body to sleep during irregular hours as you try to match the time zone of your destination.

- Keep yourself very hydrated. Because of the shifting nature of your biological clock, you can never tell when your body will be in a resting or active state. Whatever state that maybe, you need to be sure there is plenty of water in your system. Since jet lag may cause a change in your bowel movement as well, it pays to stay well-hydrated during long trips so that you land with an intact stomach and a healthy glow.

These methods have been used by many professionals in the aviation industry to keep themselves healthy despite their frequent passing through different time zones.

Restless Leg Syndrome

Also known as RLS, this condition strangely finds its way as a disorder that affects your sleep.

You may be wondering how something that affects your lower appendage meddles with a good night's sleep. At the very core, RLS affects the nervous system. It creates uncomfortable sensations in the leg. These sensations vary from the feeling of something crawling up your legs, pain, pins, limpness, and even itchiness.

These sensations happen even if there's nothing actually happening in your legs. They're all in mind. Imagine these sensations happening to you as you sleep. That is how RLS affects the quality and length of your rest. People that suffer from RLS wake up in the middle of the night to move and scratch their legs even if there's nothing wrong with them.

Causes

Interestingly, RLS also serves as a symptom of other disorders and diseases. People that suffer from Parkinson's and diabetes have been known to show symptoms of RLS. Kidney sicknesses and deficiencies with iron have also been known to share space with RLS.

Some antidepressants have also been known to induce RLS, especially when taken regularly. When taken despite showing symptoms of RLS, these drugs may end up worsening the symptoms, making pain more intense and what not.

Treatment

Since RLS is connected to other diseases, treating those conditions directly contributes to easing the symptoms of RLS. This takes coordination with your physician based on what's wrong with you.

If your medication is causing your discomfort, you need to check your prescriptions and ask your specialist for alternatives that don't bring the same side-effect.

There are also cases wherein RLS sets in after you stop taking a certain medication. This is your body getting used to a now-normal routine without the assistance of your medicine.

On another note, pampering your legs a little doesn't hurt your chances of avoiding RLS when you sleep. The following tips may be done at home to help with the symptoms:

- Getting a massage. Take note that RLS is a condition of the nervous system. Your brain sends signals to your legs to feel a certain way despite the absence of any stimuli. Feeding your nerves, a relaxing massage is one way of curbing the tendency of feeling pain. It's hard to trick your legs into feeling pain when they're relaxed and pampered.

- Hot and Cold Packs. This choice depends on your plans for the following day. If you're aiming for a cool night's rest, a cold pack for the legs is a great way to lower your temperature for the night. If you're already suffering from leg pains before going to bed, a hot pack will help blood circulation to bring more oxygen to your lower regions.

Narcolepsy

If there are disorders that cause you to avoid and disrupt sleep, there are also orders that make you sleepy when you're not supposed to be. One such example is narcolepsy.

Characterized by being excessively sleepy during the day, narcolepsy plagues 1 out of 2000 people in the United States. It may sound like a rare disorder, but it's one that doesn't just affect your day. It affects your nights as well.

People who suffer narcolepsy are almost devoid of active function. Despite having the right amount of sleep, they still become very lethargic during the waking hours of the day. They tend to fall asleep easily in the afternoon, despite there being no chance to sleep well. They may even fall asleep right in the middle of certain activities.

For patients with narcolepsy, their bodies can't really distinguish when it's time to be awake or resting. That line has been blurred. This is why they exhibit symptoms of sleepiness when they're supposed to be out and about.

On top of these problems, when they wake, their bodies can't really recognize when it's time to rest. This causes them to wake up in the middle of the night, supposedly to do something. These disruptions in their sleep and wake cycles center on an anomaly inside your hypothalamus.

Causes

The main culprit behind narcolepsy is the absence of a certain chemical produced by the brain known as hypocretin. Think of this as the "wake up" substance in the body.

When the hypothalamus creates hypocretin, the body is led to believe that the time for resting is over, and it is time to increase brain activity, metabolic rate as well as heart rate. These things are what keeps us up in the morning after we get a good night's sleep.

For a person with narcolepsy, either their hypothalamus is damaged or is not functioning properly, causing it to fail to produce this important chemical. Without this chemical, the body has no way of knowing when it's time to kick it into high gear or just to keep things mellow and sleepy.

Treatment

Sadly, narcolepsy is similar to RLS in the sense that there hasn't been a proven cure to rid someone of the disorder entirely. The delicate nature of the hypothalamus makes it hard to cure.

Despite that, there are some methods to alleviate the symptoms and to provide better energy throughout the day.

- Forcefully boost your metabolism. If your body is incapable of distinguishing awake and sleep time, you can jump-start things on your own by drinking plenty of water during the day. This will force your body to kick up its processing speeds to meet the demands of your day. About 16 ounces will do the trick

- Engage in cardio workouts. What better way to tell the body that it's time to be up and about than by giving your heart a literal run for its money? Engaging in an exercise that elevates heart rate is a great way to keep yourself alive and awake and enthusiastic during crucial parts of your workday.

- Avoid processed foods. Since your body has a sleeping metabolic rate, ingesting food that takes time to digest is only going to make things hard for you. You'll end up with clogged arteries and other disorders to complement your narcolepsy.

- Change your multivitamins. The good thing about vitamins is that you can change them depending on your need. You don't just need a simple boost of vitamin C every day. Sometimes, you need iron as well. Speak to your doctor about vitamins that boost your energy and keep you up when it is most needed.

Delayed Sleep Phase Disorder

Most commonly found in teens, this disorder stems from an abnormality with your circadian rhythm. Your body's natural metabolic rate and energy levels peak and drop at inappropriate times.

For people that suffer from this, they find it impossible to sleep in the wee hours of the morning. This is much different from a "night person" that just likes staying up late. These are people that cannot go to sleep because their bodies won't let them.

This is more of a problem with the circadian cycle of a person. It is not in sync with the body, causing a great delay in the things that are supposed to happen. People who suffer from this feel sleepy and ready for bed in the morning because of these delays. When everyone needs to go to bed, they feel like their day is just about to start.

Causes

This problem could be caused by an unhealthy development of bad sleep hygiene. Getting used to unusual hours of waking and sleeping could cause your body to adjust accordingly, changing its whole circadian clock to accommodate your unusual sleeping behavior. When this adjustment has been solidified, it becomes even harder to overcome.

This is why this disorder is seen in mostly teenagers because of their natural tendencies to stay up late. Despite that, it can also happen to adults given the proper conditions. When this happens, a solidified circadian clock with wrong bearings becomes difficult to change without drastic lifestyle changes.

Treatment

One of the best methods for restoring the circadian rhythm to normal is the use of natural light. This is also known as Bright Light Therapy.

As the name implies, the method uses artificial light to coax the body into making changes. It's a circadian clock in order to follow a normal routine. It's also called phototherapy. Here, patients go about critical portions of the day with a device called a lightbox. This box emits a bright light that emulates the brightness of natural light from the outside.

With the help of a specialist, you will be subjected to this box at certain times of the day; ideally, you want these times to be regular waking hours. Since the body follows a different cycle from the norm, the light emitted by the box will serve as a strong reminder to the body to stay active.

During sleeping hours, when it is time to rest, the lightbox is not used. When done consistently, your body will start to build a dependence on the light from the box, changing peaks, and dips in your alertness levels. During times without the box, the body will get ready for sleep.

By sticking with the therapy, you can "reset" your circadian clock and restore your sleeping habits to normal.

Fortunately, bright light therapy is also used to remedy many other types of circadian clock disorders.

Chapter 6: Consequences of Not Getting Enough Sleep

Many assume that not getting the right amount of sleep will mean being tired the following day but that with the coffee you can compensate for the sleep or catch up on sleep later when you have more time.

The problem with that approach is that the consequences of sleep deprivation are huge. Let's explore what happens to you when you fail to get the minimum amount of required sleep.

Diabetes

A 2007 study published in the Sleep Medicine Review found that sleep deprivation triggers an increased risk of diabetes in multiple ways. This link can be difficult to draw since diabetes is connected to obesity. The fact is a shortage of sleep impacts the body's ability to handle glucose. This is an important point to note.

Lack of sleep triggers so many other problems. It is difficult to distinguish the negative effects of sleep deprivation and the negative effects of triggers themselves. Whatever the case, by getting more sleep, you can decrease the various risks at the same time.

Heart Issues

Sleep plays an important role in reducing stress hormones in your system. Those hormones can damage your blood vessels and trigger high blood pressure or hypertension. High blood pressure can lead to heart disease and death.

This is an important lesson. If you want to have a healthy heart, you need to ensure you are getting enough sleep. That means planning to get more sleep. Your life may depend upon it.

Depression

The hormones that go out of balance when we lack sleep are involved with our energy and mood. When we get less sleep, we experience a negative change in mood. Some people get more sensitive and irritable. This may trigger us to be sad and overreact to negative circumstances in our environment. Depression is a high price to pay for doing something else instead of sleeping when we ought to.

Loss of Concentration

Our ability to concentrate decreases when the brain is tired from the night before, this means we will use more time to complete tasks at work and home. The quality of our work will be substandard. Clarity of thought and focus is most important when trying to get a task done quickly and accurately. When the brain is less focused, everything takes much more time.

Hallucinations

Another symptom of sleep deprivation is hallucinations. I can attest to having hallucinations. A long time ago, I was taking a trip. I had been driving for sixteen hours straight. Upon looking up, I saw a giant rabbit crossing the road. It jumped off the road before I got to it, but this was the first time I recall hallucinating.

In addition, I recall seeing lines on the road swerving as the hypnotic pattern of the reflectors on the road hit my eyes. I have since created a rule of not driving more than eight hours per day and never driving after 10 pm. Ignoring this rule could cost my life or someone else's.

Increase in Psychological Problems for Children

A Norwegian study found that children with sleep issues sometimes later develop anxiety and depression problems.

It is difficult to know what triggers what. However, it is possible to say that there is a clustering of these issues. The best way to deal with these problems is for children to get adequate sleep.

Paranoia, Anxiety, and Irritability

People are often edgy when they are sleep deprived, and they perceive risks that aren't real; they are annoyed by their environment in a manner that is not normal.

Irritability is common when people are sleep deprived. Everything around them seems annoying. Sadness is common also. For this reason, it is unwise to attempt problem-solving when sleep deprived. It is best to postpone making big life decisions until sleep is regulated. This would also be true of telephoning people, sending emails, and texts.

Skin Damage

As little as one night without sleep can lead to puffy eyes and skin issues. Chronic sleep deprivation can make these issues permanent. The elasticity of the skin can be damaged, and lines on the face can remain even after you start getting sleep. The reason for this is that fatigue triggers the body to produce the hormone cortisol, which breaks up the skin proteins responsible for keeping the skin elastic.

Inability to Learn

There are two ways in which sleep deprivation creates problems with learning:

- Impaired Short-Term Memory

- Inability to Learn Even with Repetition

People who do not have adequate sleep experience impaired short-term memories. This is seen in trying to recall things learned the day before. When a person isn't getting sleep, they struggle to remember.

Repeating a task will help a person remember. However, if the person first does the task while sleep deprived, they will find it harder to remember that same task even with repetition. This is true even when the person has enough slept the night before they attempt the task. When tired, the brain learns doesn't properly.

These two issues are important for students whose job is to learn, and yet they often suffer sleep deprivation.

Forgetfulness

A lack of sleep will prevent you from learning new information. The problem doesn't stop there. This shortage of sleep affects your ability to remember what you have learned. People who are sleep deprived find they become much more forgetful than their peers who are getting the sleep they need.

Poor Decision Making

This consequence can be expensive. It is much easier to make poor decisions when sleep deprived. In fact, people become much more willing to take bigger risks when short on sleep.

Increased Sensitivity to Pain

People who experience a lack of sleep are much more aware of pain. This is a good reason for getting enough sleep. The opposite is also true. If you have been experiencing pain, getting more sleep will help you handle the pain.

Weight Gain

The body produces two hormones that are impacted by a lack of sleep. One is called leptin, which controls a person's appetite. The other hormone is ghrelin, which makes a person want to consume more food. A shortage of sleep, even a single night, is enough to cause a decrease in leptin and an increase in ghrelin. The result is that the person is hungry and will eat more.

Weakened Immune System

If you aren't getting adequate sleep for as little as a single night, your immune system will lose its ability to fight off microorganisms. There is a connection between getting the appropriate quantity of sleep and your body's defense against bacteria and viruses.

Reduced Sex Drive

Men and women both experience a decrease in libido because of sleep deprivation. The body becomes exhausted, and the brain loses focus and desire. For men, there is a reduction in the testosterone levels triggering the drop in sex drive.

Headaches

Another common side-effect of sleep deprivation is headaches. The group hit the hardest are the people who already suffer from headaches. In particular, people who get migraine headaches can expect to increase the intensity and duration of their headaches when not getting enough sleep.

Drop-in Reaction Time

Our ability to react to situations that demand our attention decreases with a lack of sleep. This includes driving a car while tired. Many studies have shown the similarities between driving while intoxicated and driving while sleep-deprived. The similarities are so close it should be illegal to drive when lacking sleep. The problem is the inability to test whether a person has had enough sleep the night before.

Death

Although this isn't common, it still makes the news every year when people die after staying awake for days playing video games. Sleep deprivation is a life-threatening condition that should be taken seriously. Your life may depend upon how seriously you take it.

Problems with Vision

This problem can manifest itself in several ways, including dim vision, tunnel vision, or even double vision. It poses a risk when the person is driving a car or trying to accomplish something where vision is essential.

The Sum of Them All

One thing that should be clear is that the consequences of not getting enough sleep are terrible. The combination of these different issues creates a synergistic effect in amplifying the negatives.

It would be bad enough if these consequences hit you one at a time. That isn't how it works. Once you get into the habit of cutting your sleep short, you will experience several problems that trigger more problems. Sometimes it is difficult to figure out which problem is caused by lack of sleep since they all show up at the same time.

Chapter 7: Stress Can Cause Many Sleep Issues

Stress is a huge factor when it comes to insomnia. Stress can make it hard for us to fall asleep at night, and it can make it very hard for us to stay asleep if we are able to fall asleep.

Every person is going to react to stress differently. Some people may end up sleeping all of the time when they are dealing with a lot of stress. This is because they are trying to avoid their problems by simply avoiding what is making them feel stressed. Other people are going to have a hard time falling asleep because the only thing that they can think about is their problems. They may end up overthinking whatever is causing them stress, which is only going to cause them to have to deal with more stress.

Stress causes us to go into the fight or flight response. Our bodies and minds become hypervigilant or always on alert. This causes us not to be able to relax. When we go into the fight or flight response, our body responds by releasing cortisol. As we already learned, cortisol is known as the stress hormone. Too much cortisol in the body can do a lot of damage.

Because cortisol levels remain high all of the time instead of lowering at night as they are supposed to, we find that we are unable to sleep.

Stress Management

When we are dealing with a lot of stress, it can seem as if we have no control over the situation. This is what leads us to feel overwhelmed and causes us to suffer from insomnia due to stress.

Feeling that there is nothing that you can do about the stress that you are facing in your life is perfectly normal. Our bills are going to continue coming, we are never going to feel as if there are enough hours in the day to get all of the things done that we need to get done, our families and our jobs are going to continue to demand our attention, and our to-do lists are going to continue to get longer.

Believe it or not, you do have some control in these situations. Simply realizing that you are in control of your own life is going to help you to begin managing your stress so that you can start sleeping at night.

Managing your stress is all about taking control of your life through the lifestyle that you live, taking control of your thoughts as well as your emotions, and learning how to deal with problems better.

It does not matter how much you have to deal with in your life or how much stress you have. There are things that you can do in order to regain control of your life and reduce the stress that you have to deal with on a regular basis.

It is very important for us to learn how to manage our stress because when we live with constant high levels of stress, we are putting our physical and mental health at risk. Too much stress reduces our ability to function in day to day life, think clearly, or just enjoy life in general.

When we learn how to manage our stress, we break the hold that it has on our lives. This allows us to not only be healthier but happier as well as more productive. Our goal should be to learn how to balance our lives. We have to find time for our work, to focus on our relationships, to take care of all of our responsibilities, and to relax as well as have fun. We also have to learn how to deal with the pressure that we are going to face that is not planned for and face the challenges that show up in our lives.

When it comes to stress management, there is not one single thing that I can tell you to do that is going to work for every person. This is because the stress that we all face is very different in all of our lives. What may cause one-person stress may not cause another to. While one person may be stressed in one area of their lives, another person may be dealing with stress in another area of their lives.

This means that while some of these tips may work for you, some of them may not. Don't be afraid to try them all and figure out what works best for you in your situation.

1. Start by identifying the source of the stress that you are dealing with in your life. If you are dealing with stress in just one area of your life, you will want to identify that area. For example, if you have recently changed jobs, if you are moving, if you are having problems in your relationship, or if you are having financial issues.

   Understanding where the stress is coming from is very important if you want to learn how to manage it.

   It is very easy to overlook the things that are causing us stress in our lives. We tend to forget that we are people too and expect so much out of ourselves that we may not realize where the stress is coming from. If this is the case, take a look at what is going on in the different areas of your life. For example, are you not cleaning your house as you should? Perhaps you are not meeting your deadlines? Is there one area of your life that you are always procrastinating in?

   If you find that you are regularly struggling in one area of your life, this could be the area that is causing you stress. On the other hand, you may be struggling in one area because another area is demanding so much of your time. Take an honest look at your life and determine where the stress is coming from.

2. Decide what you can take control of. While there are things that you cannot control, for example, how your in-laws behave or the way that your boss acts at work, there are things that you can take control of. You can control how you will react to certain situations, how productive you are going to be, how you are going to spend your time and how you will spend your money.

It is important for you to be able to decipher what you can control and what you cannot control. The worst thing that you can do for your stress is to try and take control over things that you have no control over. If you try to do this, you are going to fail, and that is only going to cause you to feel more stressed.

Once you have determined what is causing you stress, you need to focus on the things in those specific areas that you can control. This is the best way for you to determine what action you will need to take in order to reduce your stress. For example, if you are dealing with a lot of stress because of the number of responsibilities that you have at home, try talking to your partner about it and handing some of the responsibility over to them.

Stress can make us feel as if our power in our lives has been taken away. When we focus on the things that we can change, we are taking some of that power back.

3. Do the things you love. Find something that you love to do and spend time doing it. It is easy to allow one area of our lives that we are dealing with a lot of stress to take over the rest of our lives. However, taking the time to do something we love will help us manage those other areas that are causing us stress. Doing something that you love is going to allow you to take your mind off of the things that are stressing you out, which will result in your body being able to relax. This will lead to much better sleep.

4. Learn how to manage your time. One of the biggest reasons that people find themselves over-stressed is because they do not feel as if they have enough time to get everything done that needs to be done. They have a to-do list that is a mile long, but it seems that there are not enough hours in the day to even work on it.

    Why is it that some people seem to be able to do everything? They excel at their jobs, have a side gig, are great parents and partners, their house is always clean, their bills are always paid, and they always look great? It seems that there are people out there who have more time than other people do. The truth is that we all have the same 24 hours in each day. It is up to us what we do with them. There are plenty of people out there who are sleeping 7 to 8 hours a night and still getting everything done that they need to get done while having time for their family, friends, and fun.

Take some time and write down everything that you do in one day. Don't write down things that you want to do or that you do not normally do. Be honest with yourself, and only write down what you actually do. Write down the number of hours that it takes you to do them.

On another sheet of paper, write down each hour of the day, leaving some space between them, starting with the time that you get up and ending with the time that you go to bed. Now write in all of the tasks that you do at the time that you do them, blocking out the amount of time that it takes to do them. For example, if you work from 8 a.m. to 4 p.m. every day, block that time out just for work.

How much time is left where there is nothing written? Most people will find that they have a lot of time left when they thought they had none at all. The reason that this happens is that we end up wasting a lot of our time.

Have you ever considered how many hours each week you actually sit scrolling through social media on your phone? Or how many hours you sit playing games on your devices? What about the number of hours each week that you spend watching television? All of this time adds up. Even if it is just 30 minutes per day per activity that is still 90 minutes, for just these three activities, how many other unproductive activities are you taking part in each day?

Think about the other things that you could be doing instead of wasting your time. You could be spending time with your kids at the park, going to the gym, hanging out with your friends, or even working on that project that you wanted to finish.

When we take control of our time, we often find that we have time to spend doing the things that we love, and that is going to help reduce the stress in the other areas of our lives. When we spend time doing what we enjoy, we are going to find that the thing that is causing us stress does not cross our minds. This gives our minds a break and allows them to rest, which will lead to better sleep.

5. Prepare for the stress that you are going to face in your life by knowing how you are going to handle it. Deep breathing is a great way to destress when you are standing in the grocery store checkout line, and the person in front of you seems to be taking 10 times longer than they should. However, there are times when deep breathing isn't the answer. Perhaps the answer is writing out the problem as well as all of the solutions, managing your time better. Knowing how you will manage difficult situations is going to help reduce the stress in your life, and as we have already learned, this will lead to better sleep.

6. Decide what you are going to do, what can wait, and what someone else can do. I understand if you are one of those people that would rather do everything on their own because that is the only way that you will know for sure that it is done the right way. I am one of those people. One thing that I have learned is that you can't do everything on your own. Sometimes you have to decide what you are going to do and let other people pick up the slack. You shouldn't feel as if everything is your responsibility.

If you are working 7 days a week, taking care of the house and kids when you come home, preparing all of the meals, paying all of the bills, and doing all of the grocery shopping when you are at home, your stress level is going to be so high that you are not going to be able to relax. Choose the things that you are going to do each day. If you don't have time to prepare all of the meals, delegate that task to someone else. Have someone do laundry while you shower at night or have someone do the dishes after dinner while you help the kids with their homework.

Not only is this going to help you get a little more free time, but it is going to take all of the stress off of your shoulders.

No one should have to carry the weight of the world on their shoulders, and that includes you. Look for things in your life that are causing you more stress than they are worth. Do your kids really need to do 4 extracurricular activities? Do you really need to volunteer 3 times a week? What can you do in order to reduce the number of things on your plate?

Often times, we find that we are the biggest cause of our own stress. We think that we can take on so much more than we can handle. We have to remember that we are only human. If you are doing more than you would expect from anyone else, perhaps it is too much. It might be time to start cutting back.

7. Are you opening yourself up to more stress? When we don't take the time to take care of ourselves, we are opening ourselves up to more stress. Of course, this is going to lead to less sleep, which will circle around again, leading to more stress. Are you getting enough exercise, or are you sitting on the couch all of the time? Are you skipping meals in hopes of using that time to get things done around the house? Do you have more projects going than you can handle? Are you too stubborn to ask for help?

   All of these are going to open us up to more stress in our lives, which is going to affect our health. Too much stress can cause many different physical health problems as well as mental health problems. It can cause us to suffer from insomnia. If you are leaving yourself open to more stress, you have to start taking action right now in order to stop.

8. Set boundaries. If you are the type of person that has a hard time telling people no, the chances are that you are under a huge amount of stress. I used to be that person, but let me tell you what I learned. Over the years, I learned that as long as you keep giving people are going to keep taking. If you keep allowing them to demand your time, they are going to keep demanding of your time.

At some point, you have to put your foot down and say, "Enough is enough." You have to start putting yourself first and stop taking on everything that everyone else wants you to do.

One thing that I have learned about being productive and living a happy life is that I have to focus on what is going to make me happy in my life. I cannot focus on what is going to make everyone else in the world happy. Of course, my family's happiness goes along with my own because if they are not happy, I could not be happy. As for everyone else, their happiness is their own responsibility.

I know that this may sound cold, but at some point, we have to stop trying to please everyone and decide that we are important enough to be happy as well. Saying no is going to take a lot of stress off of you. It is going to give you the time that you want to spend with your family or to do all of the fun things that you want to do.

You are not being mean by saying no, and you are not letting someone down. You are taking a stand for yourself and saying that you are important too. Trust me, someone else will always be there to say yes, so don't feel like no one is going to be there to fill the void.

Chapter 8: How to Create the Perfect Room to Sleep

Your environment plays a monumental role in affecting your different behaviors, decisions, moods, and life in general. This holds the truth for your sleep routine as well. If your sleep environment, aka your bedroom is not conducive to a good night's rest, that may be the reason why you do not sleep well at night. Here are a few practical changes you can bring to your sleep environment today to start sleeping better:

1. Dim the Lights in the Room before Going to Bed

Studies show that a dark environment actually helps trigger your sleep faster than one with glaring lights. If you sleep with all the lights switched on in your room, dim them a little now. Keep one low light on when you hit the bed to sleep as a dark environment relaxes your brain and activates the alpha waves. These slow, calm waves help you unwind and initiate sleep quickly.

Also, invest in blackout shades and heavy curtains to block out light coming in your room from the windows, so you do not wake up before your rising time and sleep well throughout the night.

2. Check the Room Temperature

If your room is too hot or too cold, that may be the reason why you keep tossing and turning on your bed the entire night. You cannot sleep when you feel hot or even when your toes are too cold. Experts suggest that temperatures between 60- and 75-degrees Fahrenheit during the summers are good enough to enable you to sleep well.

If you live in a hot country or during the summer season, make sure your room is well ventilated, so you don't feel too hot and wake up feeling exasperated. Also, invest in an efficient cooling and heating system that keeps the temperature of your house well-regulated year around promoting a good night's sleep.

When it is hot, use a fan or air conditioner to keep the air nice and cool, and if you can open a window, please do to allow fresh air into the room.

As for the chilly winters, keep your room warm enough so you stay cozy throughout your sleep. Use a central heating system to regulate the room's temperature, wear a couple of layers and use a comfy blanket to stay warm during your sleep.

3. Keep Your Room Calm and Quiet

If you sleep in a noisy room or have loud noises coming into your room during the night, that explains why you fail to sleep well. Before going to bed, ensure you switch off all sorts of noisy appliances or anything that creates even a low but constant noise because that can really get to you while you sleep.

In addition, if you have noisy neighbors, request them to keep it down during the night. You can also invest in noise cancellation installations in your house walls to block the noise coming off from the surroundings. Moreover, if you have a pet who has a habit of making loud noises throughout the night or in certain instances, keep him or her out of your room.

4. Invest in Comfy Bed, Mattress, Pillows and Bedspreads

Sometimes a hard bed or an uncomfortable mattress or pillows that are too high or a bedspread that feels itchy can keep you from drifting off to sleep easily at night. Pay close attention to your bed, mattress, pillows, and bedsheets, if any of these feel uncomfortable to you, it is time to invest in some new, super comfortable ones.

Get a bed size according to your physique and sleep needs. If you like to move around on your bed and are plus size, and sleep alone, it is best to invest in at least a Queen size bed instead. However, if you and your partner sleep together, invest in a nice Queen or King size bed so both of you can sleep comfortably on it.

As for your mattress, it needs to support your spine and legs properly. If it feels too stiff against your bed or you completely fall inside it, and it is too soft, you are likely to experience back problems in a while, which will get in the way of your good night's rest. Replace the mattress with a nice, comfy one. If you want a mattress that offers pressure relief, body contouring, and great spinal support, get a memory foam. However, if you want a nice bouncy mattress that is cool to sleep on and offers great comfort, a latex one may serve you well.

Similarly, the coiled mattress offers great support and bounce, too. You can purchase this if it suits your body well. However, some people also complain of experiencing back problems because of coiled mattresses and prefer latex ones to them. If you wish to have a softer bed, invest in a pillowtop mattress as it comes with extra cushioning.

Moreover, make sure to buy a nice, soft bed linen for your bed. Choose a material according to the season because certain materials work well only in certain seasons and can feel too warm in summers. For instance, silk and wool covers are suitable for winters, whereas cotton is more appropriate for summers but works fine year around as well.

As for your pillow, it needs to be just 3 to 4 inches in height and must be soft enough for you to lie on. If it is too hard, it may be the culprit behind your stiff neck and constant headaches and obviously, a lack of sleep. Bring these changes to your bed, and you are likely to snooze easily.

5. Leverage the Power of Natural Light

Natural light is a great way to improve your sleep-wake cycle and keeps your internal clock ticking off healthily. If there is no adequate light in your room, that may be another reason why you have an unhealthy sleep-wake cycle and sleep as well as wake up at odd hours.

While it is important to close the blinds when going to sleep, keep one slightly open so you allow natural light to flow in when the sun rises and leverage its power to help you wake up comfortably. With time, this will improve your sleep-wake cycle allowing you to sleep early and rise on time as well.

6. Change the Position of Your Bed

The position of your bed plays quite a role in determining the quality of your sleep. If it is right beside the door and your partner keeps waking up throughout the night to move in and out of the room or has a sleep routine and work timings different from yours, it can be the reason why you have interrupted sleep daily.

Also, if your bed is close to the wall adjacent to the kitchen or a noisy room or right in front of a large window in your room, it can be another reason why you fail to sleep well at night. Naturally, when noise keeps disturbing you while you struggle to sleep or a huge gush of light falls on your face early in the morning, way before your rising time, you are unable to sleep.

In these cases, it is best to change the position of your bed and move it to a quieter nook in your room to sleep better. As you bring these changes to your sleep environment, make a few to your sleep routine and habits to promote better sleep at night.

Chapter 9: Choice of Bed and Pillow

Get The Right Bed, Sheets And Mattress

Choosing the right mattress to sleep requires that you know your budget, your sleep position, and understand your own physical conditions that may interfere with your ability to sleep.

- Know the Type of Mattresses You Like – If you like a bed with some bounce to it, you'll need to choose an innerspring mattress, while if you like a firm mattress, you'll want to choose memory foam. If you like something that offers both, you can choose an innerspring mattress with a memory foam topper. Some mattresses are filled with air, like the Sleep Number bed made famous by night-time commercials and the bionic woman; this allows you to control the firmness of the mattress along with your partner.

- Know Your Sleeping Style – Believe it or not, the position you like to sleep in matters in terms of the type of mattress and pillows you buy. For example, if you want to sleep on your side, you may need an innerspring over a foam mattress because it may lessen the pressure points you feel on your hips and shoulders. If you sleep on your tummy, you will need a firmer mattress too, because you don't want to suffocate inside a soft memory foam option.

- Sleeping Temperature – If you tend to be a hot sleeper, it's essential to be mindful of this when choosing a mattress. Many memory foam mattresses have a reputation of warming up quite a bit and causing people who are hot sleepers to be even hotter. If you really want a memory foam, but you're a hot sleeper, find one of the newer "cooling" options.

- Dealing with Allergies -- If you have allergies to dust, pets, or the environment, finding a mattress that doesn't add to it is very helpful. Memory foam is antimicrobial, as well as resistant to dust mites and mold. Innerspring mattresses will need to be covered with an allergy-resistant cover to help avoid the same problems. If you do have sensitivities, you'll also want to check whether your choice is certified regarding different materials.

Don't choose something as important as a mattress on the spur of the moment. Give it a lot of thought and go to real stores to try out a mattress before ordering. Try to purchase mattresses that offer a long return option so that you don't waste your money. A good mattress should last between five and ten years.

Know your sheets (cotton, flannel, etc.). Natural fibers, meant to breathe and wick away moisture, are the most comfortable and healthiest fibers to sleep on. There are many finishes to natural cotton sheets, like sateen, t-shirt, and flannel, to name a few. If you can, avoid 100 percent polyester sheets.

Strive for 100 percent cotton or as close as you can get to it. Satin sheets have a high polyester content. I would avoid them. (Besides, they're too darn slippery!)

It used to be the higher the thread count, the higher quality of the sheet. But, wouldn't you know, when companies learned that fact impressed consumers, they started the "my thread count is higher than yours" game. SO, here's the scoop: Thread count isn't as important if polyester is a component. The length of the cotton "staple" or originating fiber is the mark of a good sheet. If a sheet is marked "Egyptian long-staple", "pima" or "supima", it is woven from a better, longer fiber. Egyptian cotton has been established as the finest of cotton materials with its characteristic longer threads. Don't buy sheets with less than a 200-thread count. They won't last.

The other benefit of buying cotton sheets without polyester is that they get softer and cozier the more often you wash them. If you are on a budget, consider getting sheets from any one of a number of surplus places that sell higher-end sheets for less than retail. (You know who they are ..., Tuesday Morning, Marshalls, Home Goods, Costco.)

Oh! And, if you are highly sensitive to finishes and dyes, consider purchasing a "pure-finish" sheet. This is a sheet that has not been finished with chemicals or dyes.

Choosing A Pillow

How many choices are there when it comes to pillows? It turns out ... many! From size to shape to stuffing, pillows are crazy complicated. Way more than they should be. My guidance? Find out what works for you.

I prefer feather or down pillows. Others prefer hypo-allergenic fiberfill. King-size or standard? Preference only. I believe more natural fibers and stuffing create a more comfortable experience. (By the way, to clean feather or down pillows, put them in the dryer for 30 minutes on high. It kills the dust mites.) Some people use memory foam. I don't particularly care for the off-gassing and VOCs (volatile organic compounds) that are part of the memory foam experience.

Chapter 10: The Best Bedtime Routine Do's and Don'ts

One way to ensure more restful night-time sleep is to set up a bedtime routine that works for you. Here is a few bedtime do's and don'ts that you may want to consider as you set yourself up for better sleep.

Do: Stop Electronics Two Hours Before Bed

So many people like watching movies before bed, but the truth is, falling asleep to movies and technology is counterproductive when it comes to ensuring a good night's sleep. Turn off your electronics at least two hours before bed and focus on low-tech, quiet activities at that point.

Do: Create A Quiet Environment

Now that you've shut down technology, it's time to quieten down the environment. While you do need to turn off your technology, it's okay to listen to a little slow and calming music in the background two hours before bedtime. However, you want the environment quiet once you lay down to sleep.

The music at the end of the day shouldn't be anything energizing or that you want to sing along with, though. The point is to create a quiet, calming environment. Maybe listen to nature sounds if you cannot take silence yet. You really do want to work toward silence two hours before bedtime.

Do: Take A Warm Bath Or Shower

Most people in today's hard-working environment tend to shower in the morning before work. It helps with the hairstyling and other factors, but the truth is, bathing before bed is a lot more beneficial to a good night's sleep. In many cultures, like Japan, it's a tradition to soak in a warm bath before bed.

A warm bath gets all the germs, pollen, and other environmental contaminants off you. Also, a warm bath or shower can be very relaxing for your muscles and help you sleep. You don't have to wash your hair to take a warm bath before bed. You can still do that in the morning if you prefer.

Don't: Use Caffeine Before Bed

Using caffeine after about 2 pm is not going to help most people sleep better. Avoid it permanently if you can, but if you can't, at least avoid it after 2 pm. If you are having issues with insomnia, you may need to stop.

Try other types of drinks that don't have caffeine. For example, if it's cold where you are, instead of sipping on hot tea, try using just hot lemon water. You'll still be warmed up, but you won't be adding anything to your digestive tract to make sleeping harder.

Don't: Drink Alcohol Before Bed

Likewise, you should not drink alcohol before bed either. Try not to have any type of alcohol after 6 pm as it can interfere with your circadian rhythm. Even if you think you're sleeping better due to the relaxation, you're not.

If you like to drink wine with your meal, that's okay, but if you find that you have insomnia, you may have to eliminate alcohol from most of your days. Everyone reacts differently to alcohol, but most people will benefit by giving it up before bed.

Don't: Drink Liquids Before Bed

One of the worst offenders in getting a good night's rest is getting up to pee. If you want to avoid this, make sure you use the toilet right before you get into the bed, but also avoid drinking any liquids at least one hour before bedtime.

Don't allow yourself to be dehydrated before bed to avoid getting up each night, though. Ensure that you mind your hydration all day long so that you don't need anything right before bed that will require you to get up.

Do: Optimize Your Bedroom

Turn your bedroom into a sleeping sanctuary. Get the best mattress you can afford as well as the best window treatments, sheets, pillows, and so forth. When it's all designed to help you relax and get more sleep, you will get more sleep.

Make your bedroom an oasis for sleeping and relaxation. When you do this, you'll notice the moment you go inside your room that you start to feel relaxed. The colors of paint you choose, the bedding you pick, and the mood you set all make a big difference in the quality of your sleep.

Do: Set Your Bedroom Temperature Cooler

If you don't have an air conditioner in your bedroom yet, you may want to consider investing in one for your wall or window, depending on where you live. Keeping your room temperature between 60 and 68 degrees is optimal for the best high-quality sleep.

Not only is setting the temperature colder good for helping you sleep, but it's also helpful to your body overall –

helping you get over colds and allergies and encouraging proper hormone production.

Don't: Eat Two Hours Before

Just like drinking can interfere with sound sleep, so can eating. You don't want to go to sleep hungry, but you also don't want to sleep when you are still digesting food. Try to limit food two hours before bedtime at the minimum to avoid needing to get up to use the toilet or other issues.

If you find that you are feeling hungry right at the two-hour mark, go ahead and have a tiny high-protein snack such as a slice of cheese or a handful of nuts, so that you don't experience hunger while trying to fall asleep. But aim not to eat closer to bedtime than that.

Do: Get Relaxed

Set up your environment so that the last couple of hours of the evening are dedicated to relaxation. That's when you can take your night-time bath, enjoy a good read while curled up in your fluffy robe, and maybe even do a little meditation, to set the mood in your mind to relax and get rest.

Make that last two hours before sleeping a relaxing time for you and your entire family. Keep your voices down, keep the lighting dim, and make everything focused on relaxation.

The most crucial aspect of your night-time routine is that you should ensure it is focused on the main point, which is to sleep soundly at night as long as possible so that you allow your body to regenerate itself in the way it is meant to each evening.

Chapter 11: Choosing the Right Foods for Sleep

The food you eat can affect the quality of your sleep. You need to pay attention to what you are eating and drinking. You might think that alcohol relaxes you, for instance. On the contrary, it actually disrupts your sleep. Find out what ingredients are in the food that you eat and choose your food wisely. You have to watch your diet not only for your health but also for the quality of your sleep.

Foods That Inhibit Sleep

There are several food ingredients that you must absolutely avoid. Caffeine, taurine, and tyramine are just some of the examples of sleep-inhibiting ingredients. These ingredients can stimulate the brain and boost adrenaline production. Keep away from the following foods and drinks.

1) Coffee – Caffeine is at the top of the list of substances to avoid if you want to improve the quality of your sleep. Coffee has loads of caffeine and should be avoided, especially near your sleep time. Drinking coffee, however, is not the only way through which you can get caffeine. Some drugs, soft drinks, tea, chocolate, and cocoa also contain

caffeine. When caffeine is ingested in high levels, it can block the bodily chemicals responsible for inducing sleep. When you drink coffee in the morning, it is not the hot temperature that stimulates your senses. Although a hot cup of coffee can make the internal temperature of the body go higher, it is the caffeine it contains that sustains alertness that is necessary to keep the body and the mind energetic. Long after the hot temperature is gone, the caffeine is still at work. Caffeine enters the bloodstream through the small intestines. Within 15 minutes, it starts stimulating the body. Its effects persist several hours after this. Studies show that the body retails half the amount of caffeine even six hours after drinking coffee or eating any foods that contain caffeine. The effects of caffeine can still be felt up to 18 to 24 hours from ingestion. If you observe that you are particularly sensitive to caffeine, try to reduce your intake of coffee and other caffeine-rich foods. If you can, try to avoid it altogether.

2) Energy drinks – In today's busy times, many people often turn to energy drinks to get that extra boost to get you going. If you are really concerned about getting an energy boost, you need to focus on improving the quality of your sleep. Cut down on

your intake of energy drinks. These drinks contain substances, primarily taurine and caffeine, which stimulate adrenaline production and activity. It is time to cut down on energy drinks. They can supplement your body with energy. That's good, but the ingredients in these drinks powerfully boost adrenaline production and activity. Taurine itself is a catalyst for natural chemical reactions in the body. When combined with caffeine, this nutrient is known to help in improving mental performance. But experts have found that such an effect is only temporary and short-lived. Just like caffeine, taurine remains in the body long after it has been ingested. Check whether the energy drinks and foods you are consuming contain this ingredient. As a guide, remember that the recommended daily consumption of taurine is 500 mg daily. Some energy drinks contain 1000 – 2000 mg.

3) Foods that contain acids – Highly acidic foods cause disturbances in the chemical composition of the stomach. As a result, you can experience heartburn, acid reflux, and other digestive problems. When you eat foods like pizza, tomato sauce, chili, and spicy foods close to bedtime, you are bound to be awakened and pulled from your sleep by gastric rumblings and discomfort caused

by an acidic stomach. Avoid acidic fruits like lemons, apples, oranges, and guavas, among others.

4) Smoked and preserved meats – The slices of ham, sausages, and bacon are looking too good to resist on the antipasti platter at dinner or on the cold cuts and cheese tray in the evening cocktails. Indulge in these foods, and it's almost a guarantee that you will be awake later than you should be. These food items are rich in the amino acid called tyramine, a brain stimulator. For meats, tyramine is produced as they undergo fermentation and/or aging. Other foods that are rich in tyramine include smoked fish, some types of beer, aged cheese, red wine, soy sauce, yeast extract, miso soup, aged chicken liver, some kinds of cacti, coconuts, Brazil nuts, peanuts, raspberries, red plums, figs, eggplants, pineapple, bananas, avocados, snow peas, beans, green bean pods, sauerkraut, tempeh, tofu, teriyaki sauce, sour cream, shrimp paste, yogurt, and chocolate. Tyramine triggers the brain to release an amino acid called norepinephrine. Norepinephrine is an understudy for the possibility of it causing migraine headaches too. Many people experience such symptoms after eating tyramine-rich foods in big amounts. This amino acid is also responsible for the headaches and hypertension in some people.

5) Chocolate – If you are a chocoholic and just cannot stop eating chocolates, you simply have to choose the lesser evil. This means choosing white chocolate versus dark or milk chocolate. Dark chocolate variants contain the highest amounts of caffeine and another brain stimulant called theobromine. Interestingly, the same substance has been found to be dangerous to cats and dogs. These animals cannot metabolize theobromine easily. For humans, theobromine causes sleeplessness and increases the risk of heart disease. If you really cannot really resist chocolates, you'll be safer with white chocolate, a variant that doesn't contain theobromine. Also, white chocolate contains a minimal amount of caffeine.

Foods To Eat For A Good Night's Sleep

There are food ingredients that can help you get to dreamland faster. A perfect night's sleep is induced with chemicals like tryptophan that help the body produce melatonin. Here are some of the best foods to eat if you are working on improving the quality of your sleep:

1) Fish – Provided that it is not smoked or dried, fish like tuna, halibut, and salmon can promote sleep. It is because fish is high in vitamin B6, a substance that's needed for the body to produce

melatonin. Melatonin can also be sourced directly from some foods.

2) Jasmine Rice – Jasmine rice has been found to have a high glycemic-index (GI). Experts said that Jasmine rice increases the amount of insulin in the blood, a condition that is conducive to tryptophan production. The higher the amount of tryptophan that gets in the brain, the faster a person falls asleep.

3) Tart Cherry – Tart cherry is rich in melatonin. In one short study involving adults suffering from chronic insomnia, the quality of sleep among these people was improved when they started consuming two cups of tart cherry juice during the daytime.

4) Yogurt – Studies suggest that being deficient in calcium can make it difficult for one to sleep. Consuming milk, yogurt, and other dairy products are recommended for improved sleep. These contain high amounts of calcium. Enriched bread, waffles, and grains, fortified soymilk, soybeans, fortified orange juice, corn flakes, raisin bran, dark leafy green vegetables, sardines, and cheese are also recommended to increase calcium intake for better sleep.

5) Whole grains – Eat more of bulgur and barley. They contain huge amounts of magnesium, another nutrient found in studies to be lacking in people who struggle with falling to sleep. You can check out the Journal of Orthomolecular Medicine if you want to get more information about how magnesium helps people sleep better.

6) Bananas – Bananas are some of the best sources of potassium. One of its other components that are often overlooked is Vitamin B6. As mentioned already, this vitamin is necessary for producing the sleep-inducing substances. Another good source of Vitamin B6 is chickpeas.

Chapter 12: 5 Exercises for Better Sleep

The exercises you'll learn can be used individually, or you can do them as a sequence, it doesn't matter as long as you do them correctly. It's possible you will fall asleep in the middle of one of them, but hey, no problem with that, right?

#1 Short Workout

If you have trouble sleeping, this quick workout can be very helpful. You can incorporate these exercises in your nighttime ritual, and, in a short time, you'll see the difference.

Exercise

1. Sit down on the floor and cross your legs. Breathe normally and regularly.

2. Now, place your elbows on top of your knees and close your eyes. Focus in on your breathing; feel how the air comes in through your nose, hold it for two seconds and exhale slowly, very slowly through your mouth. Don't force your breathing; let it flow naturally and slowly.

3. Still, in the same position, incline your trunk forward, relaxing your head. Breathe normally, regularly, and just relax. Stay in this posture for a couple of minutes and then return to the initial position.

4. Extend your legs and try to touch the tip of your toes with your hands. Relax your body, doesn't matter if you touch your toes or not, just stretch your back and relax.

5. Now, sit on top of a pillow. Any pillow as long as you feel comfortable. Keep your back straight. Use a tennis ball to massage the arch of your foot. Roll the ball back and forth under the arch of your foot.

#2 Relaxing Exercises

This is a progressive relaxation exercise, and the truth, it's amazing! You have to memorize the routine, and it can take some days to do it, but once you learn it, you'll see how your body softens, and the tension in your muscles disappears. Another thing you could do is record yourself saying this whole routine with a soothing and calming voice, and then you can listen to it at night.

Exercise

1. Lie down in your bed, find a comfortable position, and close your eyes.

2. Breathe normally; feel your feet; center your attention on your feet. Be conscious of how much they weigh, relax your feet, and feel how they sink in your bed. Start with your toes and then move to your ankles.

3. Feel your knees; center your attention on your knees. Be conscious of how much they weigh, relax your knees, and feel how they sink in your bed.

4. Feel your legs and thighs; center your attention on your legs and thighs. Be conscious of how much they weigh, relax your legs and thighs, and feel how they sink in your bed.

5. Feel your abdomen and your chest; center your attention on your abdomen and your chest. Be conscious of how much they weigh, relax your abdomen and your chest and feel how they sink in your bed.

6. Feel your buttocks; center your attention on your buttocks. Be conscious of how much it weighs, relax your buttocks, and feel how it sinks in your bed.

7. Feel your hands; center your attention on your hands. Be conscious of how much they weigh, relax your hands, and feel how they sink in your bed. Start with the thumb and continue with the rest.

8. Feel your arms; center your attention on your arms. Be conscious of how much they weigh, relax your arms, and feel how they sink in your bed.

9. Feel your shoulders; center your attention on your shoulders. Be conscious of how much they weigh, relax your shoulders, and feel how they sink in your bed.

10. Feel your neck; center your attention on your neck. Be conscious of how much it weighs, relax your neck, and feel how it sinks in your bed.

11. Feel your head; center your attention on your head. Be conscious of its weight, relax your head, and feel how it sinks in your bed.

12. Feel your mouth and your jaw; center your attention on your mouth and your jaw. Relax your mouth and pay special attention to your jaw. Feel how your mouth and your jaw sink in your bed.

13. Feel your eyes; center your attention on your eyes. Notice if there's tension in your eyes, consciously relax your eyes and feel how this tension moves away from your eyes.

14. Feel your cheeks; center your attention on your cheeks. Notice if there's any tension in your cheeks, consciously relax and move any tension away.

#3 Breathing & Sleeping Exercises

Breathing is one of the functions with more influence over your body, and breathing means life! However, it is something so natural and automatic that we never think of it as a solution. Breathing can be controlled consciously, and by doing it, you can diminish stress and help treat insomnia and many other sleeping disorders.

With basic breathing techniques, such as abdominal breathing or diaphragmatic breathing, you can reduce muscular tension and eliminate anxiety.

Exercise

1. For this exercise, you can be lying down in your bed, or however you feel comfortable.

2. Now, place one hand over your abdomen and the other hand in the upper part of your chest. This way, you can feel the diaphragmatic movements better.

3. Start by breathing in deeply and slowly, imagine the route the air makes inside your body, try to visualize it. You will note how the air reaches your stomach and how this "inflates." The thorax should not move. Contain the air inside for three seconds.

4. Relax any tension in your body; focus on your body. If your mind wanders to thoughts or worries that's ok, just bring your attention back to your body.

5. Exhale slowly while you count from five to zero and focus on every move. Notice how each time you exhale air and you feel more and more relaxed.

6. Repeat this exercise five times.

Important Note

It's important to remember to control the speed of your breathing as well as the quantity of air you inhale. Always follow a slow and paused rhythm. If you inhale too quickly or too much air you can get dizzy. If this happens, rest for a few seconds and then continue with the exercise.

#4 Getting Creative

If you are doing these exercises as a sequence, you should be feeling very relaxed by now. But if you're just getting started and some thoughts are invading your mind, then try this.

The idea of this exercise is to focus your attention on a story or a picture in your mind so you can let go of anything that is worrying you.

Exercise

1. Visualize a scene or a story, whatever you choose as long as it's calming. For example, imagine a day on the beach, a walk in the park, or a place where you feel relaxed; the idea is to find something to focus your attention on, so you let go of your thoughts.

2. Be creative, visualize every detail, try to feel the smells, see everything in your mind's eye, and let go of your thoughts. If your mind drifts to an unpleasant or worrying thought, don't fight it, acknowledge it and then let it go and continue doing your thing.

3. I'll give you an example of how it should be, but once you get it, be creative and go to your favorite place in the world, the one in where you feel most relaxed.

4. Breathe in deeply and exhale slowly. Breathe in and out, very slowly. Do these two more times.

5. Imagine you are in a big meadow; it's huge, and everything is green. You are lying down in the grass, and when you look up, you see a magnificent, clear blue sky. The sky is marvelous, and there's not one cloud in it.

6. Feel the smell of a sunny day, feel the light rays of the sun warming your face. Feel the air caressing

your face, feel the sensation of a pleasant and wonderful day.

7. Breathe in deeply and exhale slowly, enjoy every second of this. Use all of your senses to get inside this picture. It's just you and the sky...

8. Stay inside your "secret place" as long as you need to, forget about everything else and enjoy this time with you.

This is an excellent and powerful exercise; you can do it after your breathing exercise, after the progressive relaxation, or individually.

Exercise

1. Place your hands behind your head and relax. Breathe normally and regularly. Don't hold your breath.

2. Now, with your thumbs close your ear canal. Do it by placing the thumbs in the ears.

3. Hear something? You might hear a rushing sound, and if you do hear it, this means you are doing it right.

4. Stay in this position for about fifteen minutes, just listening to this sound.

5. Put your hands on your sides, breathe in deeply, and exhale one time. Relax your hands and sweet dreams!

Chapter 13: Sleep Scripts

Now that you are ready to fall asleep take a deep breath. Exhale slowly and expel any tension that may have built up during the last few exercises.

As you settle in for sleep, you may begin to have thoughts about what you have done today or things you need to get done tomorrow. Take another deep breath and let those thoughts go with your exhale. At this moment, all you need to do is clear your mind. Today is over, and tomorrow will come whether you worry about it or not. For now, clear your mind so you can wake up strong and healthy for your duties tomorrow.

For now, I want you to draw your attention to your body. Where did you store your tension today? I invite you to focus your attention on the tension and let it go as we practiced. Feel now where your body is relaxed. Take a few moments to appreciate the sense of relaxation your body is feeling at this moment and allow it to spread through your whole body from head to toes.

Before you drift off to bed, let's fill your mind with peaceful images. By promoting positive mental images, this will help you relax and can help avoid nightmares. As we begin, I would like you to visualize a place where you feel safe and comfortable. Take a few moments and imagine how the place would be.

When you have a safe place in mind, I would like you to start to relax your body again. In order to get rid of nightmares, you will need to release all tension from your body. When we are fearful, this can create tension in our bodies. Try to pay special attention to your shoulders, hands, back, neck, and jaw. Often times, these are areas where our tension can creep in.

If you feel any of these areas tensing up, focus your attention here. Breathe in...and breathe out...choose to relax and soften these areas. As you breathe, imagine the air bringing total relaxation to these areas and allow the tension to leave your body. I invite you to continue this pattern until your breathing becomes deep and slow again.

Notice now how your body has become more relaxed than it was before. Feel as your muscles sink into the bed as you relax further and deeper. Your jaw is becoming loose. Your mouth is resting, and your teeth are slightly apart. Now, your neck is relaxing, and your shoulders are falling away. Allow this to happen and let your muscles become soft.

I want you to return to your safe place. Imagine that this place is spacious, comfortable, and filled with a positive light. In this place, you have nothing to worry about, and you have all the time in the world to focus on yourself.

In this safe place, I want you to imagine the sun streaming in. The light fills you with warm and positive emotion. There are windows where you can see the beautiful nature outside. Your space can be wherever you want it to be. It can be by the mountains, by the ocean, or perhaps even on a golf course.

Return your focus back to your safe place. Imagine how warm and comfortable the room is. Walk over toward the comfortable bed and imagine how wonderful it feels to sink into the sheets. The sun is shining down on you, and you feel relaxed and warm. The bed is so soft around you, and you feel so at peace at this moment.

Notice now how these peaceful thoughts begin to fill your mind. They are filling your conscious and are clear. Any other thoughts you had before are drifting away. Your mind is falling into a positive place as you feel yourself drifting away. The space around you is safe, peaceful, and beautiful.

Any other thoughts you have at this moment, pass through your mind and drift off like clouds drifting by. Allow these thoughts to pass without judgment. There is no sense in dwelling on them when you are in such a safe place. All you have at this moment is peace and quiet.

Any time a worrying thought arises, you turn your focus back to your safe place. In this location, you can get rid of any stress you may have on a daily basis. You are here to relax and enjoy this moment. There is nothing that can bother you. You are free from stress and responsibilities here.

When you are ready, you feel your body begin to drift off to sleep. You are beginning to slip deeper and deeper toward the land of dreams. As you feel your attention drift, you are becoming sleepier, but you chose to focus on counting with me. As we count, you will become more relaxed as each number passes through.

We will now take a few breaths, and then I will count from the number one to the number ten. As you relax, your mind will drift off to deep and refreshing sleep. Ready?

Breathe in…one…two…three…and out…two…three.

Breathe in…one…two…three…and out…two…three.

Breathe in…one…two…three…and out…two…three.

Wonderful. Now, count slowly with me…one…bring your focus to the number one…

Two...you are feeling more relaxed...you are calm and peaceful...you are drifting deeper and deeper toward a wonderful night of rest.

Three...gently feel as all of the tension leaves your body. There is nothing but total relaxation filling your mind and your body. At this moment, your only focus is on quietly counting numbers with me.

Four...picture the number in your mind's eye. You are feeling even more relaxed and at peace. Your legs and arms are falling pleasantly heavy. You are so relaxed. Your body is ready for sleep.

Five...you are drifting deeper. The sleep begins to wash over you. You are at peace. You are safe. You are warm and comfortable.

Six...so relaxed...drifting off slowly...

Seven...your mind and body are completely at peace. You have not felt this calm in a while...

Eight...everything is pleasant. Your body feels heavy with sleep.

Nine...allow your mind to drift...everything is floating and relaxing...your eyelids feel comfortable and heavy...your mind giving in to the thought of sleep.

Ten...you are completely relaxed and at peace...soon, you will be drifting off to deep and comfortable sleep.

Now that you are ready to sleep, I will now count from number one to number five. All I want you to do is listen gently to the words I am saying. When I say the number five, you will drift out of hypnosis and sleep comfortably through the night.

In the morning, you will wake up feeling well-rested and stress-free. You have worked on many incredible skills during this session. You should be proud of the hard work you have put in. Now, it is time to sleep so you can wake up in the morning feeling refreshed.

Chapter 14: Meditation for Sleeping

The word "Meditation" is very popular nowadays, but most people do not know what meditation actually is? Some believe that this is a kind of mental exercise; some believe that meditation is a concentration practice.

The first thing you must know is what meditation actually is. In a very simple way, meditation is nothing but a standby mode of mind. Let me explain with a simple example: when the television or laptop is in standby mode, the power supply is continuous, current flows inside, but the television or laptop is not working, there's no picture on the screen, it's completely black. We can say it's hibernating but not shut down. In the same way, during meditation, your mind is not actively working. No thoughts, no images, no ideas, no imagination, only the power supply is on. This means you are alive, but there is a blackout in your mind. To achieve that state of mind, meditation techniques are required. Meditation techniques are just a medium to achieve a thoughtless mind, and our ultimate aim is to reach a thoughtless mind.

Preparation For Meditation

Step by Step Procedure to Prepare Yourself for Meditation:

- Lay down in bed and look at the ceiling.

- Relax your body.

- Breathe slowly – slowly.

- Be aware of the thoughts which flow through your mind.

- Let the thoughts flow. (Don't stop and don't try to divert your mind.)

- Your work is to look at the ceiling until your thoughts slow down continually.

- After a few minutes, you can easily see the ceiling without any thought.

- It will take five to ten minutes but relax.

Now, your body and mind are prepared for meditation.

Sleep Meditation

First, lie down on the bed on your back, keep your feet straight, put both hands onto the bed, and keep them straight.

Look skyward, and slowly close your eyes and focus on your breathing.

Start breathing slowly... very slowly.

Breathe in............breathe out...............

Slowly inhale...... then exhale ....

Breathe in.........breathe out...........

While inhaling, your lungs will bloom, and your chest will rise. Hold your breath for a couple of seconds, and then exhale slowly. As you breathe out, the air will slowly emerge from your lungs, and your chest will go back down.

This will help you slow down the flow of thoughts in your mind: Repeat these steps ten to fifteen times, but do remember to do it very slowly so that you can relax your body and prepare your mind for the journey of the deep, silent sleep.

Be aware of your body. Be aware from the bottom to the top of your body, head to toe. Talk with your body and say, "relax." Feel that relaxation message flowing from your mind to every part of your body, making your body relax.

Now start concentrating on the toe of your left foot. Say relax to the toe, talk with the toe, and feel the residual tension release from your toe. Feel the relaxation on your toe, now slowly move to your sole of the left foot. Release the tension from your sole and the arch of your foot. Relax them and then slowly start moving towards your heel. Release the tension from your heel, make your heel relax, and feel the relaxation.

Your toe is completely relaxed, and your sole is completely relaxed.

Now slowly move up to your ankle and release the tension from the joint of the ankle and relax the joint. Move towards the top of the foot's plane and release the tension from every muscle and make it relax.

Now concentrate on your left foot. Every muscle of your left foot is completely tension-free and relaxed...

You can talk with your body parts and say, "relax" and convey the message to your left foot and feel that your left foot is completely relaxed.

Now slowly move upward to your left leg and concentrate on shin and calf of the left leg (the shin is the top part of the leg between the knee and ankle, and the calf is the back part of the leg between the knee and the ankle).

Release the tension from the muscles and relax them, then feel the relaxation.

Now slowly move to your left knee and release the tension from the knee and relax the joints of the knee and say, "relax" to your knee.

Then, concentrate on the whole bottom part of the leg. The whole bottom part is completely relaxed. All tension from the bottom leg will be gone now.

Now move from the knee to your thigh slowly. Relax every muscle in the thigh and then move upwards to your hip and release the tension from your hip. The hip is a core part of tension because we spend too much time sitting in an office chair, so relax the muscle of your hip and say "relax" to the hip.

Now concentrate on your whole left leg. Every muscle of your left leg is tension-free, and it is completely relaxed from toe to hip.

Now, start concentrating on the toe of your right foot. Say "relax" to the toe, talk with the toe, and feel the residual tension release from your toe. Feel the relaxation on your toe. Now slowly move towards the sole of your right foot, release the tension from the sole and the arch of the sole, relax them. Then slowly start moving towards your heel. Release the tension from your heel, make your heel relax, and feel the relaxation.

Your toe is completely relaxed, and your sole is completely relaxed.

Now slowly move up to your ankle and release the tension from the joint of the ankle and relax the joint and move towards the top of the foot's plane. Release the tension from every muscle and make it relax.

Now concentrate on your right foot. Every muscle of your right foot is completely tension-free and relaxed...

Now say "relax" and convey the message to your right foot and feel that your right foot is completely relaxed.

Now slowly move upward to your right leg and concentrate on the shin and calf of the right leg.

Release the tension from the muscles and relax them, then feel the relaxation.

Slowly move to your right knee and release the tension from the knee and relax the joints of the knee. Say "relax" to your knee.

Now concentrate on the whole bottom part of the right leg. The whole bottom part is completely relaxed. All tension from the bottom leg is gone now.

Move from the knee to your thigh slowly. Relax every muscle of your thigh and then move upward to your hip and release the tension from your hip. Relax the muscles of your hip and say "relax" to your hip.

Now concentrate on your whole right leg. Every muscle of your right leg is tension-free, and it is completely relaxed from toe to hip.

Move upward and concentrate on your stomach and relax your stomach. Release the tension from your stomach and naval, then move slowly upward to your chest and concentrate on your chest. At the same time, keep breathing slowly and feel that your chest is rising and going down. Do this slowly. Now release the tension from your chest and lungs and make them relax.

Move on to your back and concentrate on your back, which is in contact with the floor or bed, and still feeling tension due to contact with the bed. Move your back a little so that the residual tension can release, and it can relax.

Then move to the fingers of your left hand and relax them. Then, very slowly move to your wrist and relax it and the joint of that wrist and move toward the elbow. Concentrate on the joint of the elbow and release the tension from the joint and relax it. Then move towards your left arm and make your arm relax and slowly move to the shoulder, which is another core tension area. Concentrate on the shoulder, release the residual stress from the shoulder, and relax it.

Now concentrate and feel the relaxation of your left hand, every muscle and every part of the left hand is tension-free and relaxed.

Then move to the fingers of your right hand and relax them. Very slowly move onto your wrist. Relax your wrist and joint, then move toward the elbow. Concentrate on the joint of the elbow and release the tension from the joints, relaxing the joint. Then move towards your right arm and make your arm relax and slowly move to the shoulder and release the residual stress from the shoulder, relaxing it.

Now the bottom part of your body is completely relaxed, and every muscle is now tension-free as well.

Feel it....

Breathe slowly-slowly

Breathe in.......... breath out.........

Slowly inhale...... then exhale ....

Breathe in..........breathe out..........

Now, slowly move upwards to your throat, relax your throat, and move your jaw and tongue. Relax them. The jaw is a core area of tension, so relax the jaw and move to your face. Relax your lips, your nose, your cheeks, your eyes, your ears, and release the tension. Now move to your forehead. This is another core area of tension. Release the tension from your forehead and feel the relaxation there.

Now move to your top of the head and release the tension. Relax and cool the top of your head.

Now the tension has completely disappeared from your body and mind, and you are feeling relaxed. Breathe slowly and feel the deep relaxation of the body. Be aware that now your relaxed body is lying on the bed and feel the relaxation of your body and the calmness of your mind.

Breathe slowly. Now you are on your bed in a deep sleep. Imagine that it's very dark around you and that you can't see anything. The only thing you can see is the darkness. Imagine that the stars are twinkling in the sky. You can see the twinkling stars in the very dark sky and feel that the stars are sending energy to your body and your mind, making them completely relaxed and calm. Feel the calmness of the twinkling stars, feel the darkness of the sky, feel the darkness around you, and feel that you are falling into a deep sleep. Your body is relaxed and calm. Your mind is relaxed and calm, and at any moment you will fall asleep, into a very deep sleep, in the peaceful darkness, In the deep silence...

Chapter 15: Exploring Sleep Cures

"The main facts in human life are five: birth, food, sleep, love, and death." -E.M. Forster

Sleep cures have been intentionally written separately from the diet management and sleeping habits so that you can explore the suggestions and choose easily for yourself those that suit you. Some of these are classic home remedies that have been around for a long time. Others are newer natural alternative treatments to try.

There are synthetic treatments that can be purchased without a prescription. It is advisable to consult a physician to get professional advice before testing them on your own. To find out more about the popular sleep treatments available today, read on:

Melatonin

Melatonin is a naturally occurring hormone in the body that is produced by the pineal gland in the brain. It induces sleep by causing drowsiness and lowering the central body temperature. Normally, the level of melatonin rises from mid to late evening, and it drops in the early hours of the morning. The production of melatonin decreases as people age. Because it is a hormone, it might not be for everyone however.

Melatonin supplements are taken by mouth in the form of capsules, tablets, or liquid suspensions. They are also available in sublingual tablets and transdermal patches. It is used to treat many medical conditions. A common use is when it's used to treat insomnia by prolonging sleep. According to studies, it is safe to take in low doses for short term use of up to 3 months. But no research for long term use has provided evidence that it is safe to use beyond 3 months. Research has yet to support its use for other sleep disorders, so it should not be treated as a one pill wonder.

Side effects and Contraindications

Melatonin supplements can cause minimal side effects if taken according to a doctor's advice. Some unwanted side effects may include nausea, irritability, a decrease in body temperature, groggy feeling in the morning, and minor changes in blood pressure. It is also not recommended for those who have heart conditions, liver problems, diabetes, and autoimmune disorders. This should be taken with caution by those who regularly drive and operate heavy machinery.

Tryptophan

Tryptophan is an amino acid that promotes normal growth & development and nitrogen balance. It is derived from specific foods that contain it. It is used by the body to produce niacin (vitamin B3) and serotonin, which is a key hormone in the sleep-wake cycle. In order for tryptophan to be converted to niacin, the body needs to have enough iron, riboflavin (vitamin B2), and pyridoxine (vitamin B6).

Tryptophan is naturally available in most protein-rich foods. It is found in dried dates, chocolate, red meat, bananas, oats, milk, cheese, sesame seeds, yogurt, turkey, chicken, peanuts, eggs, fish, pumpkin seeds, sunflower seeds, soy, other types of nuts and tofu.

Tryptophan supplements are taken orally and have long been known to induce sleep, as evidenced by clinical research results in the late 1970s. It has been shown to be effective in improving the quality of sleep. It decreases the time needed to fall asleep and increases the total amount of sleep time. These desirable effects are best displayed among those with mild insomnia and those who had difficulty falling asleep. However, it is not recommended for chronic insomnia.

Side effects and Contraindications

Tryptophan supplements can cause side effects like heartburn, gastric irritation, belching, nausea, diarrhea, and loss of appetite. It is also not recommended for pregnant and breastfeeding women, and people who suffer from digestive problems, liver disease, kidney disease, diabetes, and blood disorders. Caution should also be taken by users who drive or operate heavy machinery.

5-HTP

5-Hydroxytryptophan is a naturally occurring amino acid that is part of the biosynthesis of melatonin and tryptophan. It is available in capsule form and is used as a supplement to manage insomnia. It works by increasing the production of serotonin, which helps re-establish healthy sleep-wake patterns for sufferers of insomnia. And because serotonin's metabolic processes lead to an increase in melatonin levels, it greatly helps insomniacs get their good nights of sleep. Some studies even suggest that it is better than tryptophan supplements in inducing sleep because it has very minimal to no side effects. But that is also the problem with this supplement; it has been criticized for its lack of research to back up its effectiveness.

Side effects and Contraindications

The side effects to watch out for are similar to that of tryptophan supplements. Possible side effects are heartburn, gastric irritation, belching, nausea, diarrhea, and loss of appetite. Caution should also be taken by users who drive or operate heavy machinery. More research is needed to establish these findings.

Valerian Root

Valerian root is one of the best-known natural sleep aids. The sedative root extract is available in the form of capsules, tea supplements, and even oils. It is also one of the oldest remedies around, as it has been used for its calming effects since the 1800s. According to research, it works to hasten the onset of sleep and is supported by studies. Some experts recommend taking it with a melatonin supplement to improve its effectiveness, especially among the elderly who naturally produce less melatonin.

Side effects and Contraindications

Valerian root supplements can cause headaches, morning grogginess, excitability, and even insomnia in some people. It is also not recommended for pregnant and breastfeeding women. Caution should be taken by users who drive or operate heavy machinery. This is not recommended for people who are suffering from liver or kidney disease. This should not be taken by people who are scheduled for surgery within two weeks, because it can affect the effects of anesthesia and other medications commonly used during surgery.

Chamomile Tea

Chamomile tea is also known as the nighttime tea, thanks to its mild sedative effect that has been known about for centuries. Generally considered safe, this herbal tea has a reputation for promoting sleepiness, as well as easing anxiety and depression. Two specific types of chamomile are especially noted for their health benefits: German chamomile and Roman chamomile.

Although drinking chamomile tea is a popular choice for those who want to get a good night's sleep, there are only limited studies to back up its effectiveness. Still, a warm cup of tea can help you relax your senses and is soothing, right before bedtime. Be careful not to drink too much, though, or a full bladder may disturb your sleep.

Cherry Juice

Tart cherry juice seems promising as a sleep aid. In a short-term clinical study, experts concluded that drinking two one-ounce servings of this juice improved the quality of sleep among the participants. They napped less and had longer sleep periods. They also had significantly increased melatonin levels. Note that melatonin helps in the regulation of the sleep-wake cycle.

Also, a recent study presented at the American Society of Nutrition's annual meeting affirms the effectiveness of tart cherry juice. They believe that it is indeed an effective and preferable treatment, especially for the elderly who suffer from insomnia. It is an easily recommended choice since tart cherry juice is safer than other sleep aids that have potential side effects. The researchers also found some compounds in tart cherries that could prevent the breakdown of tryptophan, which is a possible key to its effectiveness in promoting a better quality of sleep.

Pumpkin Powder

Pumpkin is known to be rich in vitamins A and B. But recently, the seeds are becoming popular as a natural food supplement in order to help people sleep. Pumpkin powder is derived from ground pumpkin seeds. They are known to contain high levels of tryptophan, which improves the onset of sleep. In particular, the World Health Organization advocates the consumption of pumpkin seeds for its high zinc content. Aside from maintaining growth and development, immune support, and male sexual function, zinc contributes to the production of serotonin and melatonin, two important neurotransmitters that help establish the sleep-wake rhythm in our brains. It is also a rich source of magnesium, which contributes to proper blood flow and the production of energy. It contains antioxidants that promote cell rejuvenation and recovery.

Pumpkin powder is indeed a potent ingredient with many benefits in addition to inducing relaxation and sleep. It is preferred not only as a natural cure over prescription pills for insomniacs but also for its many other health benefits. According to some experts, pumpkin powder is best taken with carbohydrates to increase its effectiveness. The simplest way to ingest it is to mix one or two teaspoons of pumpkin powder in warm milk and drink it about an hour before bedtime.

Recently, pumpkin powder promoters are coming up with organic supplements that are available in powder and snack bar forms. Some of them have created a flavored powder that can be mixed with water. These are relatively new in the market at this point, so only limited clinical testing has been done. Even so, many people are buying these products in health stores as a means to alleviate insomnia.

Supplements can be used to manage insomnia. They work differently for everyone. Again, it is wise to consult your trusted medical practitioner before you decide to take any of these. Natural and safe alternatives are becoming more preferred by people for their effectiveness without the side effects.

Magnesium

Magnesium is a mineral that is powerful for helping to fight stress and anxiety. It helps relax tight muscles, calm the nervous system, and reduce pain. It also helps regulate blood sugar levels and blood pressure.

It is believed that the majority of people are getting insufficient quantities of magnesium in their diets. Even a small lack of magnesium can affect sleep quality. An effective way to improve your sleep is by adding magnesium-rich foods into your diet. Some good ones are pumpkin seeds, wheat germ, almonds, and green leafy vegetables. See medical advice. However, before taking the supplement form, as it may interact with medications you may currently be taking.

Chapter 16: Tips to Improve Sleep

1. No More Exercise Just Before Bedtime

Exercise is very important to maintain a healthy body and lifestyle, but it is important not to exercise immediately before bed. Ok, so it is true that exercise wears the body out. However, it also causes adrenaline to course through the body and sharpens the mind and also results in the body temperature to rise. Think of the time when you may have embarked on some type of exercise and then found that you are tossing and turning at bedtime, unable to sleep. This is almost certainly caused by the time of the workout, so make a concerted effort to ensure that you never workout after late afternoon.

2. Keep Your Dinner Light

Trying to go to sleep on a full stomach is difficult. The ideal time for dinner should be no later than three hours before you decide to turn in. This meal should provide protein and healthy fats with reduced carbohydrates. Keeping this meal light should not really be a problem as you probably will not need that much fuel for the remainder of the day. The larger meals should come from breakfast and lunch as these are meals where your body needs the fuel to carry on with the daily tasks.

3. Set a Caffeine curfew or if possible, give it up altogether

One of the biggest reasons why people are unable to go to sleep is caffeine. Caffeine also has the ability to lower the quality of sleep. Those who have cut caffeine out entirely apart from the odd cup once in a while have all reported that they have slept so much better since. It is strange, how big a difference that this will make, and once you have no caffeine pumping through your body it is reported that you will begin to feel like you have actually slept for the period that you have, instead of feeling that you have only slept for a couple of hours when you have actually had treble this amount or more. If cutting the caffeine out completely fills you with complete dread, then try to cut back to just two cups a day and keep these to morning and early afternoon. Set a caffeine curfew for yourself, no later than 3pm.

4. Get Up Early

Wakey, wakey, yes, it is that time of day again! If you are looking to get to bed early and for sleep to come more naturally then start by setting your alarm for 5 AM and no pressing the snooze button, as soon as you hear the alarm get up and at it, no more snoozing just get up the minute that alarm clock goes off!

For this to actually work, you will need the ultimate self-discipline, and you must not only get up immediately as soon as that alarm goes off. This must become a habit and something that you stick to every single morning, regardless of whether you have had one hour or ten hours of sleep the last night.

If you need persuading then go for a few days on just two hours of sleep and then try to say that you have not felt sleepy or are ready for bed too early than normal, this is actually the best way to reset your sleep schedule, yes you will feel dreadful for a week, but it will enable you to start afresh.

Just be prepared that this does require the ultimate in self-discipline, far more than most would like to admit, and it is far more than some people have, but it is a real-life changer.

5. **Fix Your Bedtime and Try to Make This No Later Than 10pm**

There are divided opinions on what the best bedtime is, and whether there is a general idea or whether it really is a personal choice. However, most health and fitness experts suggest going to bed between 9pm – 10pm and there is a well-known saying "the hours of sleep that you get before midnight count for two hours after." The body in general will begin to secrete melatonin at about 9:30 pm.

6. Sleep in A Dark Room – Invest in some blackout curtains!

There is nothing that will interfere with your sleep more than too much light, and whether this is coming from an electronic device or it is light that is creeping through the curtains from the outside, light will interrupt your sleep and the secretion of melatonin. If it is impossible for you to get rid of the electronics from the bedroom or if darker curtains or close shutting blinds are not an option, then invest in a good quality sleep mask. Remember to take your sleep mask with you if you are making journeys where shut-eye is going to be key and could be disturbed by light sources.

7. Get the Room Temperature Right – Ideally 12 Degrees Celsius

As the body cools down naturally when it is in sleep mode, a lower room temperature will help to regulate sleep. Ideally, you need to switch off the heating at night as leaving it on may leave you waking during the night because you have got overheated. Even during the winter, you should leave your window open to allow fresh air and oxygen to enter the room. The ideal sleep temperature is reported to be about 12 degrees Celsius (54 F), although there are some experts that claim a temperature between 60 – 65F is ideal, this is more matter of choice so you will need to do a little trial and error to see which works best for you.

8. **Light Mental Exercises**

Many experts, including Dr. Vicky Seelall have recommended that doing light mental exercises while you're trying to sleep great for getting your body to fall into a natural deep sleep. Whether you try counting backward from 100 using multiples of three, yes challenging to ensure that you pay attention but easy enough for you to be able to remain relaxed. By partaking in these types of simple challenges, you are taking your mind off of things that could keep you awake and will lull you into a state of relaxation, and you are more than likely to find that sleep will be not too far around the corner.

9. **Finish the Day's Business in Your Mind**

Get into the habit of planning your following day before you go to bed, and this alleviates the impulse to start going over what you need to do for the following day whilst you are trying to get off to sleep. You may find that it is beneficial to write down any of the day's worries to get them off of your mind too. Get into the habit of only thinking positive thoughts prior to sleeping and celebrate your own positive successes by keeping a handy list that you can always revisit if things aren't going as well as you want them too and you need a boost to your positivity.

10. **No Over-Thinking**

Overthinking whilst you are trying to sleep will result in no sleep. This is because overthinking makes the brain active, and this is the cause of insomnia. Getting a good night's sleep is definitely linked with clear thinking and ensuring that you allow your mind to disengage with all that has gone on during the day or is currently going on in your life.

11. **Your Bedroom Should be An Electronic-Free Zone**

Taking all manner of electronic gadgets to bed with you is simply going to lead you to confuse your brain by giving it an overdose of stimulation, and then you won't sleep. Therefore, the bedroom should be a strict electronic-free zone. It will not take your brain long to understand and be taught that a bedroom is a place of rest. There is a reason Steve Jobs didn't even allow apple devices in the bedroom.

12. **Extinguish All Sources of Light & Avoid Blinking Lights**

Even the smallest of light sources can disturb sleep and sleeping patterns. Research has shown that even those that have a Mac mini in their bedroom that they use as a media player and the light on this really is tiny, and it pulsates on and off. When the mini has been switched off completely, better sleep was recorded, proving that it must have been the tiny light that was the distraction as the machine itself was totally silent. It is difficult to comprehend that it can be such a tiny light that affects sleep and quality. Try pitch black as this is really the only ideal situation for proper quality sleep.

13. **Clear Your Mind**

There is no doubt that we have all been kept awake with worries and niggles such as, did I complete the tasks needed today? What if I forget to make that call in the morning? I must hit that deadline, or I could lose the work......... and so on.

From now on, take a few minutes before turning in for the night and grab a pen and paper or your keyboard and jot everything down, sweeping all thoughts from your mind. By getting everything out of you head you will feel as though you have everything recorded and that you can use this list when you are ready to deal with the contents, this is also an excellent exercise if you are wanting to get more organized as you are in effect planning tomorrows tasks in readiness for the following day, leaving your mind clear to sleep.

Things to note down are those tasks that need completing, the people you need to contact, ideas that you have had through the day but failed to do anything with, write down everything regardless of how significant and you will be surprised how much easier sleep will become.

14. **Have A Glass of Milk Before Bed?**

It could be a case of "Mother Knows Best!" but remember when you were a child and could not sleep the majority of us will have been given a warm cup of milk or other beverage and nine times out of ten it would have worked!

Milk is particularly good for sleep; this is because it is made up of an amino acid known as tryptophan that is converted first to serotonin and then melatonin, which is known as a hormone that helps with sleep. Strangely enough, Tryptophan is also found in turkey, which is why you may feel particularly sleepy after Christmas or Thanksgiving dinner.

15. **Comfort - Pjs, Mattress and Pillows**

Spare a thought to how much time you actually spend sleeping, now think how much money you have invested in this area of your life. The majority of people will indeed buy the cheapest mattress and pillows that are on offer, and yet they are still shocked when they are uncomfortable when they try to go to sleep. The moral is that if you want a decent night's sleep, then you should spend as much as you can afford on a high-quality mattress and also pillows. If you suffer from ruin sleep and back pain, the chances are that your mattress is to blame!

Indulging and spoiling yourself with a high-end mattress that you sink into and matching pillows are the best thing after cutting out caffeine as far as sleep improvements go! Good quality nightwear is a must too, go for the pajamas that you would happily wear all day if you could and maybe on occasions you do. You should look forward to sleep and the comfort that it brings to your body.

16. Hypnotherapy or Meditation Before Bedtime

If you are looking for ways to enhance your sleep further and really take it to the following level, then meditation and hypnotherapy could be just the thing that you are looking for. Both are very similar in that they are quiet yet focus the mind. The idea behind meditation is to focus on one thing whilst hypnotherapy is you focusing on aspects of yourself that you want to improve and mentally repeating this until it takes effect.

There are several simple meditation exercises; one of the most common is to focus all of your thoughts on your breathing. A simple meditation exercise I use each night is to focus my thoughts on my breathing. Mentally note how cold the air feels whilst you are inhaling and how warm it is when you are exhaling and how your tummy expands and contracts. As your focus is purely on your breathing, no other thoughts get to enter your mind.

Try just 10 minutes of meditation before sleeping, and you will be amazed at the HUGE difference to the quality of sleep you will be rewarded with, you will feel as though you have added hours to the length of your sleep on rising the following day.

17. Sleep in A Quiet Room

OK, so it is stating the obvious to say that silence will help us to sleep. Health and fitness experts have suggested that it is not a good idea to use white noise to gain better sleep but that this should be used to drown out other sounds that may keep us awake. What works best though in the majority of cases is to keep things as simple as possible, and there is a noise outside that you are powerless to shut up, for example, car alarms or barking dogs, then get some earplugs to enable the noise to be canceled out.

On the flip side, other health specialists champion soothing sounds. However, this is really in the case of those that wake at the slightest sound. Suggestions include trying a fan in the room to create white noise or have a track of rain or running water playing in the background, and there is a new free app called Sleepmaker Rain that could be downloaded to be used at bedtime, just remember to keep that screen face down to avoid any light source.

18. Herbal Tea Before Bed

There are a number of studies that show taking a melatonin supplement will help you to fall asleep quicker, and although fine in the short term taking anything for a prolonged period of time could negatively affect your health. However, a good alternative could be drinking tea. In particular, chamomile tea has been an advocate as an herbal remedy for the treatment of anxiety, stress, and insomnia due to its calming properties. If all you need to do is have a brew before bed, then I think it's time to put the kettle on!

19. Nap Control

There are times where all you can think about is having a nap and you really just need a nap, and it could be because it is one of those really long days that seem to go on forever or that you didn't get much sleep the night before for one reason or another. Taking a nap will not affect your sleep provided that the nap is not for too long. The majority of doctors and health/fitness experts agree that a 20 – 30 minute power nap is the best way to kick start energy levels during the day. However, these naps should always be taken before 3pm or at an absolute push 4pm, any later or longer than the specified half-hour, and the person will probably experience difficulty getting to sleep in the evening. Don't fall into the trap and sabotage your great sleeping work by failing to adhere to these wise nap rules!

20.   Hack Your Body Temperature

An acclaimed sleep scientist P. Lewis has recommended that you fool your body temperature before sleep. Studies report that the body goes through a cooling process when it is in sleep mode. Therefore, there is no reason why you cannot trick your body into believing that it is going to sleep by actually raising your body temperature before going to bed. This can be achieved by having a hot bath or shower or simply by dipping your feet into some hot water. Then when you go to bed in your cooler room, your body is tricked into thinking that it is time to go to bed because it cools down in the same way as it does when you are asleep. Trying this with a combination of the other items suggested in this list could actually help you to fall asleep faster.

Chapter 17: Recommended Lifestyle for Improved Sleep and Rested Mind

The nature of our lifestyles impacts our sleeping patterns a great deal, and it is also one of the reasons why most of us have difficulty falling asleep at night. Unhealthy or sedentary lifestyles can lead to anxiety, restlessness, which in turn will cause insomniac complaints at many levels. Some find it hard to fall asleep while the others wake up easily in the night, and going back to sleep once again seems just out of the question. At times there are several factors that affect your sleep, such as work stress, hectic deadlines, pending workload, relationship issues, personal problems, and more. We might not be able to sort out everything before hitting the bed. However, some precautions will help you relax and fall asleep more easily than before. The good news is that a simple lifestyle change can work wonders in improving your sleep cycles. Read on for some common tips and suggestions to induce and ensure sound sleep:

Fix a Sleeping Schedule: Most of us tend to have erratic sleep timings or no timings at all. It might seem convenient to grab a few hours of sleep and head out or run errands or tackle chores, but over time, this untimely habit will only cause drastic effects on your health and well-being. It is a good practice to set a sleeping time and even important to ensure that you follow it faithfully. The internal system or the circadian rhythm is like an inbuilt setting in the body, which reminds us when we should sleep or wake up. When we miss the natural setting of day and night, this circadian rhythm gets totally messed up, and the body will no longer be able to decipher whether it is supposed to sleep or stay awake and alert. In order to avoid messing your body's internal default setting, fix a sleeping time, and make sure you are already tucked in and on the way to dreamland by that time. Make it a point to hit the bed and wake up at the same time every day. In case you find it difficult to fall asleep, it is a good idea to wake up and do something relaxing and de-stressing for a few minutes till you fall asleep again. Try not to stay up or distracted for too long as this will affect your sleep pattern

Eat and Drink on Time: Try to take your meals on time, especially dinner, and ensure that it is a good few hours before bedtime. You should neither feel hungry or too full before bedtime as either of these conditions will disturb your sleep. A heavy dinner will cause discomfort and keep you up for long hours, and similarly, consuming too many drinks will lead to frequent trips to the restroom throughout the night. Limit your intake of caffeine or alcohol before bedtime because the former will prevent you from falling asleep and the later, although, it might induce sleep but only to disrupt it later on. Some people are accustomed to consuming their cup of espresso before bedtime, which is highly not recommended as it can stay in the system for up to 12 hours. Take care to avoid all forms of caffeine post-lunch hour for a good night's sleep. Some light snacks such as turkey or dairy products actually help induce sleep as they contain tryptophan, which is basically an amino acid that helps your body by releasing melatonin or serotonin, which is also considered as a sleep-promoting hormone. For instance, light but delicious snack of crackers with cheese or yogurt is sufficient to do the trick.

Bedtime Ritual: Creating and maintaining a bedtime ritual is ideal because it is a way to trick your body into believing that it is time to hit the bed. The ritual can include just anything that you used to do- a warm shower, followed by a skincare or moisturizing session, a song or two, a conversation with your loved one, and so on. Stay away from late-night television or movies as this will beat all sense of timing and keep you awake and hooked to the screen beyond bedtime. In short, try to indulge in simple activities that make the transgression from being awake to a state of drowsiness easier and comfortable.

Restrict Daytime Naps: Some of us find it necessary to nap during the day, especially in the afternoons. While this habit can come as a source of great comfort, it may be a bit of a problem for all those suffering from insomniac conditions. If you are a light or poor sleeper, avoid long naps in this way, your body will feel tired and sleepy as night approaches. Sleeping during the day might keep you up and alert even past midnight. If you really need the need to nap to lay off some stress or fatigue, restrict it to 10 to 30 minutes and no more. However, these rules do not apply to someone who works at night. In cases when it's impossible to follow the natural sleep schedule, try to keep your room sleep-friendly whenever it's time to hit the bed.

Stay Physically Active: Getting your body used to being active and moving about is a good way to tire your body into a good sleep. It is highly recommended to follow an exercise routine as this will not only help you in staying fit and toned but will also keep modern-day ailments at bay. When you are physically active, your body will be able to fall asleep much easier and also enjoy deep sleep patterns. However, timing is a great thing, and care should be taken to avoid all exercises post evening as this only keeps the body alert and active, which deters sleep. Working before bedtime is a big no, so make sure to fit in an activity or two some other time of the day.

Keep Stress at Bay: One of the many enemies of sleep is stress and its related drawbacks. However, avoiding stress altogether may not always be possible, but it is always feasible to keep it at bay, especially before you retire to bed. When your mind is constantly worrying about the things that need to be done before time, your stress levels increase, and any desire to sleep is pushed to the backseat. To avoid stress from taking over your life, it is a good idea to plan and organize your list of things to be done. Set a calendar and organize your day. Make sure to get your tasks done on time and try your best to avoid procrastination. Prioritize your tasks and get them done accordingly. Delegate whenever possible, as this ensures your work is done without pressurizing yourself too much. Finally, always take out some time for yourself. Indulge in activities that help you to de-stress or rejuvenate. It can be anything like time spent with friends, a good massage, a spa day, a date with love on, a good laugh, or just anything that makes you feel alive and happy. Try to live life to the fullest, so you have no regrets to brood over and spoil your sleep. Plan your day in advance and convince yourself that what needs to be done tomorrow should be left for tomorrow. Calm yourself down and allow sleep to take over gradually.

Chapter 18: Create a Daily Routine that Helps with Sleeping

There are many things that we do throughout the day that we do without the knowledge that we might be inhibiting our abilities to sleep later in the day.

Limit or Avoid Taking Naps

If you can help it, try to avoid taking naps as much as possible during the day. Sleeping during the day can greatly inhibit your ability to fall asleep when it is time to hit the hay. If you must have a nap, limit your time to no more than 20-30 minutes. If you sleep any more than this, you may feel groggier than when you laid down to gather a small recharge in the first place.

Exercise During the Day

Exercise of all kinds is something that we should be doing every day or at least 120-150 minutes 3-4 times a week. It aids in an overall improvement of health and mainly aids in sleep by reducing the stress we tend to carry around. Try to exercise no later than 3 hours before bedtime. Otherwise, the adrenaline your body produces while exercising may actually inhibit you from falling asleep.

Watch What You Eat

Instead of a big meal of steak and potatoes before bedtime, consume a lighter meal instead. Heavy meals are much more difficult for our bodies to digest and trust me; indigestion is not fun to experience when you are trying to go to sleep. You should not go to bed hungry either, for the hunger pangs you may experience will keep you awake as well. Eat a light snack right before bedtime, such as hummus, Greek yogurt, cheese, or bananas (to name a few) to aid in better sleepy time.

Prep Your Bedroom

The place in which you catch your zzz's should be 100% free of gadgets of all kinds. Turn off the television and remove items such as laptops and phones. These items will only keep your mind too active for sleep because you are tempted to look at notifications. Your bedroom (or wherever you rest) is meant to get adequate rest, not for working or scrolling through your social media.

The lower the temperature of your room while you sleep, the better. The recommended temperature is right at 65 degrees. This helps in keeping your body temperature at a low enough number to help you fall and stay asleep.

Weighted blankets are great in keeping pressure on your body that aids in the relaxation of the nervous system that promotes a nice, deep sleep. The best weight to aim for is a blanket that is 15-30 pounds. It will feel like you are receiving a big warm hug from a favorite person, which is quite calming.

The higher quality your bedding is the better sleep you are more likely going to receive. Get a mattress that is comfortable and supports your entire body. Even though mattresses can be expensive, trust me, it is very worth the investment. Your bed is where you spend a third of your life after all! Ensure that you make your bed up with comfortable sheets and pillows as well. There are many kinds of bedding on the market. The better quality that your overall bedding is, the better your chances are to fall and stay asleep faster.

Dim the lights! As you have previously read, even the smallest of lights can greatly impact your ability to fall and stay asleep. With the help of installing light dimmers and/or wearing an eye mask, you can block out pesky lights that you may have no control over, like streetlamps.

Control Disruptive Noises

Sometimes, just shutting the bedroom door is not enough to adequately block out noises that may come from within your bedroom, a commotion outside, or from your neighbors. There are machines that are available to purchase that utilize calming white noise or ocean sounds that do a great job at keeping distracting noises at bay. Do your best not to rely on your phone to play these sounds.

Wear comfortable earplugs that you should dedicate just for sleeping time. There are many different kinds that are made up of soothing materials that are also easy to clean.

Establish Bedtime and Wake Up Times

Begin your routine that you perform for bedtime at the same time each evening. This not only helps you maintain a regular and healthy sleep cycle, but it enables your body to fall asleep faster and easier. This is the same for the time you wake up as well. Do your best on the weekends to not sleep in for more than an hour at the most. Creating good sleeping habits can make a world of difference in your overall health as well.

Read

Reading 30 minutes to an hour before bedtime or reading to fall asleep is a popular way that people can successfully shut off their brains to the day's events and engulf themselves in an entirely another world that they can think about before drifting into a deep slumber. Pick either a boring or entertaining read that helps you get rid of your mind of worries and things you need to do the following day. For sleeping purposes, stay away from self-help, DIY, or other reading material that stimulates the mind.

Practice Stretching and Relaxation Techniques

You have already become privy to some of the relaxation methods that are great ways to wind down before falling asleep. Performing yoga or gently stretching various areas of your body before you lie down, helps immensely regarding being able to fall asleep.

Utilization of Journals

I personally keep two journals, one that I write my thoughts and to-do lists down in and one that I document the dreams that I recall and take an interest in wanting to remember. Doodling and writing worrisome thoughts help you to relieve your brain in having to keep all those negative thoughts trapped within it. Jotting down dreams can help you see a pattern if you need to know of one, and for me, as a writer, it is like free creative material delivered to me via sleep that I can utilize in future pieces!

Wear Comfy Clothing

When heading to bed, ensure that you are wearing loose-fitting clothing that has the capability to stay cool throughout the night. Or you could sleep naked! This is probably the most comfortable way to sleep, for you do not have to worry about your clothing making you uncomfortable in the middle of the night or making you too warm.

Chapter 19: How to Maintain a Regular Sleep Schedule

Have you noticed how babies do not seem to have any trouble dozing off whenever they want to? Their sleep and wake time and cycle are regular. It is during this time when their body's growth processes are stimulated. When they wake up, they have boundless energy to play and entertain everyone around them. As far as their parents are concerned, these sleep patterns allow them to follow a routine. As these babies grow older, their sleep patterns change due to a number of factors. Adults often have erratic sleeping habits. As a result, the quality of sleep gets compromised. The late nights and short snooze times cause people to become sluggish and less alert.

It's not hopeless for you to revert to a healthier sleep habit. Fortunately, the body is a trainable machine. It can be trained to "sleep like a baby" to have all the energy you need to survive your days. Your first step is to train the body to follow a sleep schedule. Check out the following tips:

- Think that you can do it. It's all about attitude. Saying that you cannot do it and giving excuses like "Going to bed at an early time won't help me doze off to sleep right away," "It's not easy," or "It's just impossible for me to obtain 8 hours of sleep straight" will not get you anywhere. Don't make excuses. Tell yourself that you can do it and BELIEVE that you can do it. It takes time to develop a habit, so be patient with yourself. There are steps to help you ease into a new and healthier sleeping habit.

- Select a time range for sleeping. Determine a time frame that you want to designate as your "official" sleep time. Set a specific time when you absolutely need to be in bed already. Set the latest time that you will allow yourself to be awake at night. If you finish dinner at around 8pm, you can set 10pm to 11pm as your sleep time. Start preparing for bed an hour after this time.

Designate a wake-up time too. You can do this by adding at least 7 hours to your latest sleep time. This will be your earliest wake-up time, and your latest will be an hour after. It is advisable not to go beyond these wake-up times as well. Even if you don't feel like getting up yet, force yourself out of bed and get started with your day. You might be tempted to sleep in during the weekends, but when you are getting enough quality sleep, there will be no need to do this at all. Stick to your sleep schedule ALL days of the week.

- Remove distractions at least an hour before your appointed sleep time. These distractions are referred to as "sleep robbers" as they keep you from sleeping. They make your mind wander and keep your senses awake. The most common distractions are the TV's light radiation that creates dancing shadows on the walls, the mobile phone that beeps every once in a while, and the computer that tempts you to surf and browse all night long. These all keep the brain awake and thinking. Turn everything off an hour before you get into bed.

There are some people who get frightened or do not feel comfortable in a dark and quiet room. These feelings can be considered as "sleep robbers" too. You can have soft sounds like the hum of the air conditioner or the electric fan. You can also have relaxing instrumental music playing softly. There are CDs with audio material intended to relax you enough to make you sleep more peacefully. There are also clock radios that play soothing sound effects of nature like the rushing waves at the beach, the soft falling sound of raindrops, or the chirping sound of birds. Feel free to choose whichever sound you prefer to help you sleep better.

- Develop a sleep preparation routine. It's not only the physical aspects of your sleep environment that you have to pay attention to. After you have created the perfect sleep ambiance, you have to get your mind and body ready for sleep as well. Have a routine before you go to bed. The start of your routine will switch your mind towards thinking about sleep. Take a quick shower, brush your teeth, and do your beauty regimen. This routine gives the body the signal that it will soon have to go to sleep. Do the same things every night to condition the mind and body more effectively?

- Do not nap too close to your bedtime. When you have had a particularly tiring day, you are most likely to get tired and sleepy early. Resist the urge to take a nap late in the afternoon. It will definitely affect your sleep schedule. You cannot yield to drowsiness anytime it hits. Finish whatever tasks you can finish until you get as close to your sleep schedule as possible. Then, go through your sleep preparation routine. Get a full night's sleep and wake-up within 7-8 hours of your sleep time.

There are plenty of studies that promote the benefits of taking naps. Even the shortest nap can give you the rest that you need and reenergize your body. Just be sure to take your naps early in the day. Around midday is a good schedule for naps. It gives the body a quick rest from your morning activities and reenergizes it for the rest of the day. Sometimes, pushing on and keeping the mind and body active until bedtime is the best way to ensure that sleep comes to you during your scheduled sleep time.

Conclusion

In the broad spectrum of things, stress is the leading factor in our lives that causes further health complications from a physical standpoint in our bodies to mental impairment of our ability to focus and an emotional standpoint that disables our ability to cope with life's challenges. Stress alone causes these factors that affect our ability to sleep, but if left unchecked, it can exacerbate our health to serious illnesses and disorders that may even threaten our lives.

The cycle of feeling stressed, having our quality of sleep suffer because of it, and then continuing to suffer because of a lack of good sleep can be ongoing. In order to get substantial relief and pull ourselves out of this cycle and onto a healthy road of recovery and relaxed living, we must identify our unhealthy habits that contribute to our stressful state. After identifying them, we need to work diligently to stop them and redirect our lives by instilling healthy habits. This is not in order to be a health fanatic. This is so that we can actually feel good about ourselves, feel empowered to live our lives the way that we want to live them that keep us feeling good, and so that we can become immune to areas of our lives we once saw as stressful by changing our mental outlook.

All of these factors, in small changes and small steps, will help to ensure a permanent change in the way we feel from day to day, and as equally important, they will help us to get the rest that we so deserve. By practicing small changes in our lives to help ourselves feel more relaxed and at peace, we allow ourselves to sleep better at night. And in sleeping better at night, we will have then created a new cycle in our lives that is self-sustaining.

I hope that it has provided you with a way or a few to break your cycle of poor sleep so that you can start feeling more comfortable within yourself, more energized throughout your day, and more peaceful at night. Sleep well.

Printed in Great Britain
by Amazon

49458646R00095